S0-CBI-718

Histological Typing of Testis Tumours

Springer

Berlin
Heidelberg
New York
Barcelona
Budapest
Hong Kong
London
Milan
Paris
Santa Clara
Singapore
Tokyo

World Health Organization

The series *International Histological Classification of Tumours* consists of the following volumes. Each of these volumes – apart from volumes 1 and 2, which have already been revised – will appear in a revised edition within the next few years. Volumes of the current editions can be ordered through WHO, Distribution and Sales, Avenue Appia, CH-1211 Geneva 27.

1. Histological typing of lung tumours (1967, second edition 1981)
2. Histological typing of breast tumours (1968, second edition 1981)
4. Histological typing of oral and oropharyngeal tumours (1971)
8. Cytology of the female genital tract (1973)
9. Histological typing of ovarian tumours (1973)
10. Histological typing of urinary bladder tumours (1973)
14. Histological and cytological typing of neoplastic diseases of haematopoietic and lymphoid tissues (1976)
17. Cytology of non-gynaecological sites (1977)
22. Histological typing of prostate tumours (1980)
23. Histological typing of endocrine tumours (1980)
24. Histological typing of tumours of the eye and its adnexa (1980)

A coded compendium of the International Histological Classification of Tumours (1978).

The following volumes have already appeared in a revised second edition with Springer-Verlag:
Histological Typing of Thyroid Tumours. Hedinger/Williams/Sobin (1988)
Histological Typing of Intestinal Tumours. Jass/Sobin (1989)
Histological Typing of Oesophageal and Gastric Tumours. Watanabe/Jass/Sobin (1990)
Histological Typing of Tumours of the Gallbladder and Extrahepatic Bile Ducts. Albores-Saavedra/Henson/Sobin (1990)
Histological Typing of Tumours of the Upper Respiratory Tract and Ear. Shanmugaratnam/Sobin (1981)
Histological Typing of Salivary Gland Tumours. Seifert (1991)
Histological Typing of Odontogenic Tumours. Kramer/Pindborg/Shear (1992)
Histological Typing of Tumours of the Central Nervous System. Kleihues/Burger/Scheithauer (1993)
Histological Typing of Bone Tumours. Schajowicz (1993)
Histological Typing of Soft Tissue Tumours. Weiss (1994)
Histological Typing of Female Genital Tract Tumours. Scully et al. (1994)
Histological Typing of Tumours of the Liver. Ishak et al. (1994)
Histological Typing of Tumours of the Exocrine Pancreas. Klöppel/Solcia/Longnecker/Capella/Sobin (1996)
Histological Typing of Skin Tumours. Heenan/Elder/Sobin (1996)
Histological Typing of Cancer and Precancer of the Oral Mucosa. Pindborg/Reichart/Smith/van der Waal (1997)
Histological Typing of Kidney Tumours. Mostofi/Davis (1998)
Histological Typing of Testis Tumours. Mostofi/Sesterhenn (1998)

Histological Typing
of Testis Tumours

F. K. Mostofi and I. A. Sesterhenn

In Collaboration with L. H. Sobin
and Pathologists in 9 Countries

Second Edition

With 175 Colour Figures

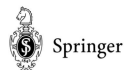 Springer

RC258
A1
I614
no.16
1998

Dr. F. K. Mostofi
Isabell A. Sesterhenn

Department of Genitourinary Pathology
Armed Forces Institute of Pathology
Washington DC 20306-6000, USA

First edition published by WHO in 1977 as No. 16 in the International Histological Classification of Tumours series

ISBN 3-540-63374-X Springer-Verlag Berlin Heidelberg New York

Library of Congress Cataloging-in-Publication Data
Mostofi, F. K. (Fathollah Keshvar), 1911–. Histological typing of testis tumours / F. K. Mostofi and
I. A. Sesterhenn, in collaboration with L. H. Sobin and pathologists in 9 countries. – 2nd ed. p. cm. –
(International histological classification of tumours) Includes bibliographical references and index.
ISBN 3-540-63374-X (softcover : alk. paper)
1. Testis–Tumours–Histopathology–Classification. I. Sesterhenn, I. II. Sobin, L. H. III. Title. IV. Series: International histological classification of tumours (Unnumbered) [DNLM: 1. Testicular Neo-
plasms-pathology. 2. Testicular Neoplasms-classification.   WJ 858 M916h 1998]   RC280.T4M67
1998.   616.99'263-dc21 DNLM/DLC   97-30424

This work is subject to copyright. All rights are reserved, whether the whole or part of the material is
concerned, specifically the rights of translation, reprinting, reuse of illustrations, recitation, broadcast-
ing, reproduction on microfilm or in any other ways, and storage in data banks. Duplication of this
publication or parts thereof is permitted only under the provisions of the German Copyright Law of
September 9, 1965, in its current version, and permission for use must always be obtained from
Springer-Verlag. Violations are liable for prosecution under the German Copyright Law.

© Springer-Verlag Berlin Heidelberg 1998
Printed in Germany

The use of general descriptive names, registered names, trademarks, etc. in this publication does not
imply, even in the absence of a specific statement, that such names are exempt from the relevant
protective laws and regulations and therefore free for general use.

Product liability: The publisher cannot guarantee the accuracy of any information about dosage and
application contained in this book. In every individual case the user must check such information by
consulting the relevant literature.

Typesetting, printing, and bookbinding: Appl, Wemding
SPIN: 10635920   81/3135 – 5 4 3 2 1 0 – Printed on acid-free paper

Participants

Cabanne, F., Dr.
Centre Georges-François Leclerc, Dijon, France

Hedinger, Chr. E., Dr.
Department of Pathology, University Hospital, Zurich, Switzerland

Jacobsen, G. K., Dr.
Department of Pathology, Gentofte Hospital, University of Copenhagen, Hellerup, Denmark

Morinaga, S., Dr.
Department of Pathology, Saiseikai Central Hospital, Tokyo, Japan

Mostofi, F. K., Dr.
Department of Genitourinary Pathology, Armed Forces Institute of Pathology, Washington DC, USA

Nistal, M., Dr.
Departmento de Morfologia, Universidad Autónoma Madrid, Spain

Parkinson, M. C., Dr.
Department of Histopathology, UCL Hospitals Trust and University College London Medical School, London, England

Romanenko, A., Dr.
Department of Pathology, Research Institute of Urology and Nephrology Kiev, Ukraine

Scully, R. E., Dr.
Department of Pathology, Massachusetts General Hospital,
Boston, USA

Sesterhenn, Isabell A.
Department of Genitourinary Pathology, Armed Forces Institute of Pathology, Washington DC, USA

Sobin, L. H., Dr.
WHO Collaborating Center for International Histological Clas-
sification of Tumours, Armed Forces Institute of Pathology,
Washington DC, USA

Teppo, L., Dr.
Finnish Cancer Registry, Helsinki, Finland

The authors thank Dr. Charles J. Davis, Jr. for his valuable con-
tribution in preparation of this publication.

General Preface to the Series

Among the prerequisites for comparative studies of cancer are international agreement on histological criteria for the definition and classification of cancer types and a standardized nomenclature. An internationally agreed classification of tumours, acceptable alike to physicians, surgeons, radiologists, pathologists and statisticians, would enable cancer workers in all parts of the world to compare their findings and would facilitate collaboration among them.

In a report published in 1952[1], a subcommittee of the World Health Organization (WHO) Expert Committee on Health Statistics discussed the general principles that should govern the statistical classification of tumours and agreed that, to ensure the necessary flexibility and ease of coding, three separate classifications were needed according to (1) anatomical site, (2) histological type, and (3) degree of malignancy. A classification according to anatomical site is available in the International Classification of Diseases[2].

In 1956, the WHO Executive Board passed a resolution[3] requesting the Director-General to explore the possibility that WHO might organize centres in various parts of the world and arrange for the collection of human tissues and their histological classification. The main purpose of such centres would be to develop histological definitions of cancer types and to facilitate the wide adoption of a uniform nomenclature. The resolution was endorsed by the Tenth World Health Assembly in May 1957[4].

---

[1] WHO (1952) WHO Technical Report Series, no. 53. WHO, Geneva, p 45
[2] WHO (1977) Manual of the international statistical classification of diseases, injuries, and causes of death, 1975 version. WHO, Geneva
[3] WHO (1956) WHO Official Records, no. 68, p 14 (resolution EB 17.R40)
[4] WHO (1957) WHO Official Records, no. 79, p 467 (resolution WHA 10.18)

Since 1958, WHO has established a number of centres concerned with this subject. The result of this endeavour has been the International Histological Classification of Tumours, a multi-volumed series whose first edition was published between 1967 and 1981. The present revised second edition aims to update the classification, reflecting progress in diagnosis and the relevance of tumour types to clinical and epidemiological features.

Preface to Histological Typing of Testis Tumours – Second Edition

The first edition of *Histological Typing of Testis Tumours*[1] was the result of a collaborative effort organized by WHO and carried out by the WHO Collaborating Centre for Histological Classification of Male Genitourinary Tumours, Armed Forces Institute of Pathology, Washington DC. The classification was published in 1977[1] and has been widely utilized with little or no modification.

In order to keep the classification up-to-date, a set of proposals for revision was circulated to the participants listed on pp. V–VI. Their responses provided the basis for a new draft. After further communications among the participants, the present classification, definitions and explanatory notes were recommended for publication.

The histological classification of testis tumours, which appears on pp. 3–5, contains the morphology code numbers of the International Classification of Diseases for Oncology (ICD-O)[2] and the Systematized Nomenclature of Medicine (SNOMED)[3].

It will, of course, be appreciated that the classification reflects the present state of knowledge and modifications are almost certain to be needed as experience accumulates. Although the present classification has been adopted by the members of the group, it necessarily represents a view from which some pathologists may wish to dissent. Nevertheless, it is hoped that, in the interests of international cooperation, all pathologists will

---

[1] Mostofi FK, Sobin LH (1977) Histological typing of testis tumours. World Health Organization, Geneva (International Histological Classification of Tumours, No. 16)

[2] World Health Organization (1990) International classification of diseases for oncology. Geneva

[3] College of American Pathologists (1982) Systematized nomenclature of medicine. Chicago

use the classification as suggested. Criticism and suggestions for its improvement will be welcomed; these should be sent to the World Health Organization, 1211 Geneva 27, Switzerland.

The publications in the series *International Histological Classification of Tumours* are not intended to serve as textbooks, but rather to promote the adoption of a uniform terminology that will facilitate communication among cancer workers. For this reason, literature references have intentionally been omitted and readers should refer to standard works for bibliographies.

Contents

Introduction

This classification is based primarily on the presence of morphologically identifiable cell types and growth patterns that can be correlated with the clinical behaviour of the tumour and, in some cases, with tumour markers in the serum. Although some of the histological terms and definitions have histogenetic implications, this classification is not meant to be histogenetic. The terminology adopted for individual tumours is based on their general acceptance and world-wide usage. Synonyms are included only if they have been widely used in the literature or if they are considered helpful in understanding the lesions. Controversial histogenetic terms have been avoided whenever possible.

The term *tumour* is used synonymously with *neoplasm*. The term *tumour-like* is applied to non-neoplastic lesions which clinically or morphologically resemble neoplasms; they are included in this classification because of their importance in differential diagnosis.

Because of the many similarities between testis tumours and those of the ovary, an attempt has been made to follow the WHO histological typing of ovarian tumours.

Histological Classification of Testis Tumours

---

[1] Morphology code of the International Classification of Diseases for Oncology (ICD-O) and the Systematized Nomenclature of Medicine (SNOMED)

**3   Tumours Containing Both Germ Cell
           and Sex Cord/Gonadal Stromal Elements**

4   Miscellaneous Tumours

5   Lymphoid and Haematopoietic Tumours

6   Tumours of Collecting Ducts and Rete

**7   Tumours of the Tunica, Epididymis, Spermatic
           Cord, Supporting Structures, and Appendices**

Definitions and Explanatory Notes

1 Germ Cell Tumours

The large majority of primary testicular tumours originate from germ cells. More than half of the tumours contain more than one tumour type: seminoma, embryonal carcinoma, yolk sac tumour, polyembryoma, choriocarcinoma, and teratoma. In over 90%, the histology of the metastasis is identical to that of the primary tumour. Every cell type in the primary tumour, irrespective of its benign histological appearance or volume, is capable of invasion and metastasis. Thus, the information provided by the pathologist guides the urologic surgeon and the oncologist towards the best mode of therapy. The report of the pathologist can explain the relationship of the histology of the tumour to tumour markers and the response of the metastasis to the specific postorchiectomy treatment. If the metastases do not respond to the treatment, they may consist of some form of teratoma for which surgical intervention is the method of treatment.

In 10% of cases, the histological features of the metastases may be different from those of the initial sections of the primary tumour. Further sectioning may identify an additional element in the primary tumour or a scar referred to as a regressed or burned out tumour, with or without intra- and extratubular malignant germ cells.

Therefore, it is essential that the specimen be examined adequately with extensive slicing and macroscopic description, including the major dimensions. Tissue available for microscopic examination must include the tumour (at least one block for each 1-cm maximum tumour diameter and more if the tissue is heterogeneous), the non-neoplastic testis, the tunica nearest the neoplasm, the epididymis, the lower cord, and the upper cord at the level of surgical resection. The specimen should not be discarded until the clinician and the pathologist have agreed that the pathology report and diagnosis correlate with the clinical features. The presence of discordant findings (e.g. elevated aFP in a seminoma) indicates a need for further sectioning of the gross specimen.

Since the WHO classification was proposed in 1977, one or more of the following markers have been used in clinical diagnosis, staging and monitoring the response to therapy: alpha foetoprotein (aFP), human chorionic gonadotropin (hCG), human placental lactogen (hPL), pregnancy-specific beta-1 glycoprotein (SP1), placental alkaline phosphatase (PLAP), carcinoembryonic antigen (CEA) and lactic dehydrogenase (LDH). The two markers most widely adopted and of greatest clinical value are aFP and hCG.

It is now recognized that in testicular germ cell tumours, syncytiotrophoblastic cells, whether they occur singly or within a choriocarcinoma, are the most common source of hCG. The cells recapitulate their development in the placenta. They occur as large or multinucleated giant cells with eosinophilic, glassy cytoplasm and large or small vacuoles which may contain erythrocytes and/or as spindle-shaped endothelial-like cells. In sections stained with haematoxylin and eosin (H + E), the syncytiotrophoblastic cells may be overlooked until highlighted with immunohistochemistry, utilizing antibodies to placental glycoproteins, e.g. hCG, hPL and SP1. hCG can be demonstrated in over 90% of morphologically recognizable syncytiotrophoblastic cells, but occasionally these cells are not stained for hCG. Although hCG production is almost exclusively seen in syncytiotrophoblastic cells, rarely it may be encountered in bizarre epithelial cells of testicular teratomatous origin.

Scattered solitary or aggregates of syncytiotrophoblastic cells are present in about 40% of testicular germ cell tumours, either intermingled with other neoplastic cell types, in the stroma or, more rarely, in the adjacent seminiferous tubules or vascular spaces. They are often associated with small foci of haemorrhage, which is a helpful diagnostic feature both macroscopically and microscopically, particularly in seminoma.

The presence of syncytiotrophoblastic cells alone should not lead to the diagnosis of choriocarcinoma, but should be listed in the diagnosis. Otherwise, the urologist may attribute an elevated serum level of hCG to other elements in the tumour.

Yolk sac tumour is the principal source of aFP, but aFP may also be present in some embryonal carcinoma cells and in enteric and hepatic cells of mature and immature teratomas.

Immunohistochemical demonstration of aFP and hCG permits correlation between pathological and clinical findings, especially when the H + E-stained sections do not readily reveal the element(s) responsible for these markers in the serum.

Post-orchiectomy persistence or an increase of serum levels of either hCG or aFP is indicative of the responsible cells in the metastases. In monitoring the course and the response to therapy, one should not interpret normal serum marker levels, particularly of aFP, to indicate an absence of metastases, especially of embryonal carcinoma.

After therapy, a metastatic deposit may show necrosis, scar tissue, persistence of a tumour identical to the primary lesion or, occasionally, the presence of another germ cell element not seen in the initial slides of the primary tumour. In some 40 % of these metastases, mature and/or immature teratoma are seen. In about 10 %, malignant tumours of the types seen in other organs, e.g. sarcomas and adenocarcinomas, are found, explaining the lack of response to the usual chemotherapy or radiation therapy.

Treatment may inhibit production of tumour markers such as aFP by viable-appearing yolk sac elements.

Rudimentary or streak gonads (generally referred to as dysgenesis), maldescent and androgen-insensitivity syndrome (AIS) are characterized by an increased incidence of testis tumours and tumour-like lesions. In patients with cryptorchidism, foci of immature seminiferous tubules often form small nodules that may be confused with Sertoli cell tumours. Cryptorchids are particularly prone to contain germ cell tumours, most commonly seminomas, which may involve one or both of the testes. Sertoli and Leydig cell hamartomas and malignant germ cell tumours may be seen in AIS.

The age of the patient provides a clue to the most likely type of tumour present. In the newborn, the most frequent testicular tumour is the juvenile granulosa cell tumour. Most germ cell tumours occur between the ages of 20 and 50 years. Before puberty, seminoma is extremely uncommon, while yolk sac tumours and the better differentiated types of teratoma are the usual germ cell tumours. Spermatocytic seminoma and malignant lymphoma usually occur in older patients, although both may also occur in younger individuals.

In addition to histological typing of the tumour, the estimated quantity of cell types, determination of vascular/lymphatic invasion and the pathological stage of the tumour should be reported. The TNM staging system is recommended (see page 35).

1.1 Precursor lesions – intratubular malignant germ cells (Figs. 1–5)

Germ cells with abundant vacuolated cytoplasm and large, irregular nuclei located within the seminiferous tubules.

The cytoplasm contains abundant glycogen and reacts positively with antibodies to PLAP. The chromatin pattern is coarse and there may be two or more nucleoli and abnormal mitoses. The cells typically form a single layer at the periphery of the tubules but may also occur singly. Spermatogenesis is usually absent in the affected tubules.

Intratubular malignant germ cells may extend along the seminiferous tubules into the rete testis where they undermine or intermingle with rete cells. This may be misinterpreted as carcinoma of rete testis, but it has no prognostic significance. Microinvasion of interstitial tissue and vascular and/or lymphatic spaces may occur. The infiltrating cells are often associated with a lymphocytic infiltrate.

Synonyms: carcinoma in situ, intratubular preinvasive tumour, intratubular atypical germ cells and intratubular germ cell neoplasia.

1.2 Tumours of one histological type (pure forms)

1.2.1 Seminoma (Figs. 6–15)

A germ cell tumour of fairly uniform cells, typically with clear or dense eosinophilic glycogen-containing cytoplasm, a large regular nucleus with one or more nucleoli and well-defined cell borders.

The appearance of the cells depends to a large extent on fixation and preparation. The cytoplasm typically contains glycogen, a feature that is helpful in distinguishing seminoma from spermatocytic seminoma and lymphoma. PLAP is uniformly positive along the cell membrane and/or in the cytoplasm of most seminomas. LDH can be demonstrated in most of the tumour cells. Cytokeratin may be positive in some cells to a variable degree; therefore, the presence of cytokeratin in a germ cell tumour does not exclude the diagnosis of seminoma. hCG, SP1, hPL and aFP are not demonstrable in seminoma cells. A characteristic feature seen in almost all cases of seminoma is lymphocytic infiltration. Granulomatous reaction may also be seen with Langhans or non-specific giant cells. Occasionally, the granulomatous reaction is so extensive that it masks the tumour cells, but their presence may be confirmed by PAS and PLAP positivity. The stroma varies in amount.

The tumour cells form irregular lobules, cords or strands. They can be arranged diffusely or, less commonly, surround irregular anastomosing spaces simulating gland formation or yolk sac tumour. Rarely, the tumour is exclusively intratubular. Seminomas with numerous mitoses (averaging 30 mitoses in 10 consecutive high power fields throughout the tumour) have been designated as *seminomas with high mitotic index* replacing the previous designation *anaplastic seminoma*.

1.2.1.1 Variant – Seminoma with syncytiotrophoblastic cells
(Figs. 16–20)

Seminomas with syncytiotrophoblastic cells should be distinguished from mixed seminoma and choriocarcinoma. Small haemorrhages are frequently associated with the syncytiotrophoblastic elements.

1.2.2 Spermatocytic seminoma (Figs. 21–24)

A tumour composed of germ cells that vary in size from lymphocyte-like to giant cells of about 100 μm in diameter, with the bulk of the tumour composed of cells of intermediate size.

These cells have eosinophilic cytoplasm and round nuclei. The nuclei of the larger cells have a filamentous or spireme pattern similar to that seen in spermatocytes. Mitoses are often numerous but metastasis is extremely rare. Oedematous or mucous stroma is reflected macroscopically by a soft, mushy texture or cystic appearance. Spermatocytic seminoma frequently also shows an intratubular growth pattern, but intratubular malignant germ cells as defined above are absent.

In about one-third of spermatocytic seminomas, isolated tumour cells contain PLAP. hCG, SP1, aFP, hPL and cytokeratin are not demonstrable.

1.2.2.1 Variant – Spermatocytic seminoma with sarcoma
(Figs. 25–26)

A spermatocytic seminoma associated with an undifferentiated or, less frequently, with a differentiated sarcoma (e. g. rhabdomyosarcoma).

The sarcomatous component may metastasize, but metastasis of the spermatocytic seminoma is extremely rare. Therefore, wide sampling of any tissue with varied macroscopic appearances is indicated. It is not, as yet, clear whether or not this should be classified as a tumour of more than one histological type (Sect. 1.3).

1.2.3 Embryonal carcinoma (Figs. 27–37)

A tumour composed of undifferentiated anaplastic cells of epithelial appearance with abundant clear to granular cytoplasm and a variety of growth patterns.

These cells are large and lack distinct borders. The nuclei are large and typically more pleomorphic than those of seminomas. They are usually vesicular with a see-through appearance, but may be hyperchromatic, particularly in frozen sections. The nuclei often overlap and have one or more nucleoli. Mitoses are frequent.

The cytoplasm is homogeneously amphophilic, basophilic or clear. aFP may be demonstrable in rare individual cells or in small groups of cells. Cytokeratin may be present while epithelial membrane antigen (EMA) generally is not demonstrable. Embryonal carcinoma cells do not contain hCG or SP1, but hPL may be present in some cells.

The stroma varies considerably: scanty, loose, oedematous, fibrous, hyalinized or quite cellular with or without lymphocytic infiltration. The presence of a cellular stroma, per se, does not constitute teratoma.

Several growth patterns are encountered: papillary, solid, glandular or tubular formation. In rare conditions, only intratubular growth is seen.

Solid embryonal carcinoma must be distinguished from seminoma. The most helpful features are less distinct cell membranes, nuclear crowding and clear nuclei in embryonal carcinoma. Although aFP and hPL are rare in embryonal carcinoma, they are absent in seminoma. Low molecular weight cytokeratin, although more strongly positive in embryonal carcinoma, is not reliable in distinguishing embryonal carcinoma from seminoma. PLAP is demonstrable in both.

In all embryonal carcinomas, it is important to search for and report on vascular and lymphatic invasion and extratesticular extension. Syncytiotrophoblastic cells may occur scattered within the tumour. Their presence should be recorded.

Synonym: malignant teratoma undifferentiated (includes yolk sac tumour in adults).

1.2.4 Yolk sac tumour (Figs. 38–54)

A tumour characterized by a loose vacuolated network of small cells forming anastomosing tubuloacinar structures and simulating yolk sac, allantois and extra-embryonic mesenchyme.

Yolk sac tumour cells have uniform, round vesicular or hyperchromatic nuclei. They are low or high cuboidal or elongated and spindle shaped. There can be marked cellular pleomorphism, particularly in adults. The cytoplasm is usually vacuolated and may contain scattered hyaline PAS positive-diastase resistant globules. Fat and glycogen are often present. The cytoplasm reacts positively with antibodies to aFP, but the distribution of aFP is generally patchy and of varying intensity. The cells may show immunoreactivity for PLAP, but none of the cells react with antibodies to hCG, hPL or SP1.

The stroma varies; it may be oedematous, myxomatous or cellular. Extracellular deposition of eosinophilic hyaline material (laminin) can be extensive. In infants and children, haematopoiesis may be present. Vascular and lymphatic invasion is frequent.

Many histological patterns occur: microcystic, macrocystic, reticular, papillary, solid, glandular/alveolar, enteric, myxomatous, endodermal sinus, polyvesicular-vitelline, parietal and hepatoid. The reticular pattern consists of a loose network of anastomosing tubuloacinar structures lined by flat, low or high columnar cells. Papillary structures with a delicate fibrovascular core and covered by low cuboidal to high columnar epithelium, known as endodermal sinus or Schiller-Duval bodies, are frequently present, but are not pathognomonic, as similar structures rarely occur in embryonal carcinoma and other tumours. Syncytiotrophoblastic cells may be scattered within the tumour and should be reported.

A solid yolk sac tumour can be distinguished from seminoma because it does not have lymphocytic infiltration. It may have laminin and hyaline bodies and, most importantly, it is generally associated with various other patterns.

Synonyms: endodermal sinus tumour, orchioblastoma, malignant teratoma undifferentiated (in adults).

1.2.5 Polyembryoma (Figs. 55–57)

A rare tumour composed predominantly of embryoid bodies.

In its fully developed form, the embryoid body is composed of an amniotic cavity, germ disc, yolk sac, extraembryonic mesenchyme and syncytiotrophoblastic cells. The structure resembles a 2-week old embryo. Differentiation may occur to form the full spectrum of teratomatous elements. In pure form, polyembryoma is extremely rare in the testis, but embryoid bodies, sometimes poorly formed, are found most frequently in association with teratoma and in mixed tumours. The polyembryoma often shows a positive reaction for hCG in syncytiotrophoblastic cells and aFP in yolk sac elements.

The term "diffuse embryoma" has been used when yolk sac elements form a necklace-like structure surrounding circles of much larger embryonal carcinoma cells. These should be classified under Sect. 1.3, *Tumours of more than one histological type.*

1.2.6 Trophoblastic tumours

1.2.6.1 Choriocarcinoma (Figs. 58–64)

A tumour composed entirely of syncytiotrophoblastic cells and cytotrophoblastic cells.

The histological appearance of syncytiotrophoblastic cells is described in Sect. 1, *Germ Cell Tumours,* p. 8.

Cytotrophoblastic cells may constitute the bulk of the tumour. They consist of sheets of small, uniform, hexagonal cells with pale eosinophilic or clear cytoplasm and regular, small, round vesicular or hyperchromatic nuclei with or without nucleoli. These cells are recognizable only by their intimate relationship with syncytiotrophoblastic cells.

Syncytiotrophoblastic cells usually form the advancing edge of the tumour and may suggest villous formation, but they can also be intermingled with cytotrophoblastic cells.

Choriocarcinomatous foci associated with other germ cell tumour types are more common than pure choriocarcinoma and should be classified under Sect.1.3, *Tumours of more than one histological type.*

Synonym: malignant teratoma trophoblastic; this includes both choriocarcinoma and any combination of choriocarcinoma with germ cell tumours other than seminoma.

1.2.6.2 Placental site trophoblastic tumour (Figs. 65–68)

A rare tumour composed of mononucleated cells with eosinophilic or vacuolated cytoplasm resembling early stages of syncytiotrophoblastic cells.

The cells have been described as intermediate trophoblasts. They react positively with hPL and occasionally with hCG and/or SP1. In most instances, the tumour occurs in association with teratoma, in which case it should be classified under Sect.1.3, *Tumours of more than one histological type.*

1.2.7 Teratoma (Figs. 69–85)

A tumour that is typically composed of several types of tissue representing different germinal layers (endoderm, mesoderm and ectoderm).

When tissues representing only endoderm or only ectoderm, e.g. skin and brain, are the only tissues present, such a tumour is regarded as a monodermal teratoma. If a single type of differentiated tissue, e.g. cartilage, a mucous gland or squamous cyst, is associated with a seminoma, embryonal carcinoma, yolk sac tumour or choriocarcinoma, that tissue is considered to be a teratomatous component. Epidermal cysts shown to be pure by extensive sectioning are not classified as teratoma. Syncytiotrophoblastic cells may occur in different categories of teratoma as in other germ cell tumours. Teratoma may produce aFP in areas with gastrointestinal and hepatic differentiation.

1.2.7.1 Mature teratoma (Figs. 69–74)

A teratoma composed exclusively of well-differentiated mature tissues.

Ectodermal elements are typically represented by squamous epithelium, with or without keratinization, salivary glands and neural tissue; endodermal structures by gastrointestinal, hepatic, pancreatic and respiratory tissue; and mesodermal elements by cartilage, bone and muscle. Mitoses are rare.

In adults, in spite of apparent maturity and benign histological appearance, mature teratoma is capable of vascular and lymphatic invasion and metastasis; these should be searched for and reported. In infants and prepubertal children, mature teratoma is usually benign.

Synonym: teratoma differentiated.

1.2.7.1.1 Dermoid cyst (Fig. 75)

A mature teratoma with a predominance of one or more cysts lined by keratinizing squamous epithelium with skin appendages, with or without small areas of other teratomatous elements.

Dermoid cysts are rare in the testis in contrast to the ovary. They should be diagnosed as such and distinguished from epidermal cysts, which are lined by keratinizing squamous epithelium without skin appendages.

1.2.7.2 Immature teratoma (Figs. 76–80)

A teratoma in which there are incompletely differentiated immature or embryonal tissues.

Foetal neuroectodermal elements, embryonal mucous glands, immature cartilage and immature mesenchymal elements are common components. Mitotic activity may be high. aFP is demonstrable in the primitive gastrointestinal glands and hepatic tissue. In adults, immature teratoma has the capability of vascular and lymphatic invasion and metastases. In infants and prepubertal children, immature teratoma is benign.

Synonym: teratoma differentiated.

1.2.7.3 Teratoma with malignant areas (Figs. 81–85)

A teratoma containing a malignant component of a type typically encountered in other organs and tissues, e. g. sarcomas and carcinomas.

The most frequent forms of this type are undifferentiated sarcoma, rhabdomyosarcoma and chondrosarcoma. The undifferentiated sarcoma of this category may be difficult to distinguish from mesenchymal elements of immature teratoma, but the latter resemble spindle cells seen in foetal tissue and are often oriented with epithelial elements in an organoid pattern. If such arrangement is not seen or atypical mitoses are present, the area is diagnosed as sarcoma. Among carcinomas, adenocarcinoma is more frequent than squamous cell carcinoma. Neuroepithelioma, neuroblastoma and nephroblastoma occur. Carcinoid in a teratoma should be classified here.

The type of malignant component is specified in the diagnosis, e.g. *teratoma with carcinoid or teratoma with rhabdomyosarcoma.*

1.3 Tumours of more than one histological type (mixed forms) (Figs. 86–93)

This category includes germ cell tumours composed of two or more types.

All components that are present should be listed in the diagnosis and their quantity estimated, as this information may be clinically significant. About 60 % of testicular germ cell tumours consist of two or more histological types. Since the syncytiotrophoblastic cell is not a tumour type, pure germ cell tumours associated with syncytiotrophoblastic cells are not included in this category.

Except for spermatocytic seminoma, which occurs almost always in pure form, the tumour types can occur in any combination. Spermatocytic seminoma with sarcoma is listed under Sect. 1.2.2.1 since the origin of the sarcoma is unknown. In tumours of more than one histological type, embryonal carcinoma, yolk sac tumour and teratoma with syncytiotrophoblastic cells are the most frequent combinations.

Synonyms: malignant teratoma intermediate includes only teratoma and embryonal carcinoma; combined tumours, malignant teratoma trophoblastic.

Any of the germ cell tumours can undergo regression resulting in a scar representing a burned out tumour (Fig. 94).

2 Sex Cord/Gonadal Stromal Tumours
(Figs. 95–115)

2.1 Pure forms

Included in this category are Leydig cell tumours, Sertoli cell tumours, granulosa cell tumours and tumours of the thecoma/fibroma group.

These tumours constitute about 4 %–6 % of adult testicular tumours and over 30 % of testicular tumours in infants and children. The name given to this group does not indicate a preference for any particular concept of testicular embryogenesis. As with the germ cell tumours, the aim throughout this section is to closely parallel the WHO terminology and classification of ovarian tumours.

About 10 % of these tumours, almost always in adults, metastasize. However, it may not be possible on histological grounds to forecast their behaviour. The criteria for malignancy are discussed in Sect. 2.1.1 below. Some of these tumours occur in AIS and should be classified under Sect. 11.3.

Synonyms: specialized gonadal stromal tumours, mesenchymomas, sex-cord mesenchymal tumours and sex-cord stromal tumours.

2.1.1 Leydig cell tumour (Figs. 95–101)

A tumour composed of elements recapitulating normal development and evolution of Leydig cells.

The most common appearance is that of medium-sized cells with distinct cell borders, eosinophilic cytoplasm and a round or oval vesicular and rarely grooved nucleus, frequently containing a prominent nucleolus.

The cells may be larger with finely or coarsely vacuolated cytoplasm containing lipids, while others consist of elongated, spindle-shaped cells with granular eosinophilic cytoplasm. The nuclei may vary from small to large, round to oval, or vesicular to pyknotic. Occasional cells may be binucleated.

The Reinke crystal is helpful in the identification of Leydig cell tumours, but is detectable in only about 40 % of cases. Lipofuscin pigment is often present. The cells occur in sheets, columns, cords and trabeculae. One of the distinguishing features of Leydig cell tumours is the delicate endocrine type of vascularity, best observed when the tumour occurs in sheets. Leydig cell tumours correspond to hilus cell tumours of the ovary.

In children, these tumours are associated with pubertas praecox. In adults, gynaecomastia and other signs of feminization may be present.

About 10 % of Leydig cell tumours are malignant (Figs. 97 100). The criteria for the diagnosis of malignancy are anaplasia of the cells, individual cell necrosis, larger areas of tumour necrosis, extension to the tunica or epididymis, increased mitotic activity and vascular invasion. However, rarely the tumour may show none of these features but still metastasize. In such cases, the metastases are usually delayed 5 or more years.

Leydig cell tumours have to be distinguished from nodular aggregates of Leydig cells found in the testes of persons with atrophy, cryptorchid, the Klinefelter syndrome and Klinefelter-like syndrome. In such cases, the testes are small and the seminiferous tubules are small and often sclerotic. Hyperplasia differs from neoplasia in that the tubules are entrapped in the former but not in the latter; although a few entrapped tubules may be seen in the periphery of a tumour.

Leydig cell tumours and hyperplasia can be distinguished from similar changes in the androgen insensitivity and the adrenogenital syndromes by the absence of clinical symptoms or laboratory evidence of those syndromes.

Extraparenchymal Leydig cells, isolated or, more commonly, in groups, occur in the spermatic cord and tunica albuginea without denoting malignancy.

Synonym: interstitial cell tumour.

2.1.2 Sertoli cell tumour (Figs. 102–106)

A tumour composed of Sertoli cells typically arranged in well-defined tubules.

These tumour cells range in shape from oval to columnar. They have a small or medium-sized, round or oval vesicular nucleus containing a fine chromatin network and a solitary, small, basophilic nucleolus. The cytoplasm may be scanty or abundant with a single large or multiple small lipid vacuoles. When distended with lipid vacuoles, the tumour corresponds to the lipid rich Sertoli cell tumour of the ovary. Sometimes the tumour cells have an eosinophilic granular cytoplasm. Rarely, they contain slender Charcot-Boettcher crystalloids. Call-Exner like laminated calcified bodies may be found. The cells form tubules with a more or less distinct lumen which may contain basement membrane-like material, or the tubules appear solid as in the prepubertal testis. The tumour may occur in sheets with only occasional tubule formation. The stroma can be scanty or composed of abundant, sometimes hyalinized, fibrous tissue.

Sertoli cell tumours must be distinguished from the small nodules of coiled tubules lined by immature Sertoli cells found in over 20 % of cryptorchids and occasionally in descended testes. Such nodules are sometimes mislabeled Sertoli cell or tubular adenoma, but represent residual nodules of immature tubules. Occasionally, scattered spermatogonia are found within the tubules of the Sertoli cell nodules.

2.1.2.1 Variants

2.1.2.1.1 Large cell calcifying Sertoli cell tumour (Figs. 107–108)

A Sertoli cell tumour with large cells and calcification.

These cells are large with cuboidal, hexagonal, columnar or spindle shapes. The cytoplasm is abundant, finely granular and eosinophilic, but may be amphophilic and slightly vacuolated and contain abundant lipid in fine droplets or large vacuoles. Rarely, Charcot-Boettcher crystalloids are present. The nuclei are round, oval or elongated with one or two small nucleoli. Mitoses are generally absent or rare. The neoplastic cells often form tubules or cords, clusters, trabeculae or solid sheets. The stroma may be loose, myxoid or densely collagenous with varying degrees of calcification. Calcification appears as large, wavy, laminated nodules or massive deposits; sometimes it is sparse.

In the absence of prominent tubule formation and minimal calcification, the tumour may simulate a Leydig cell tumour, especially in a child with precocious puberty.

The large cell calcifying Sertoli cell tumour is most common in children and is often associated with hyperplasia and neoplasia of other endocrine organs, including testicular Leydig cell tumours, bilateral primary adrenocortical hyperplasia and pituitary adenomas, spotty mucocutaneous pigmentation and cardiac myxomas. Clinical associations have included sexual precocity, acromegaly, pituitary gigantism, hypercortisolaemia, Peutz-Jeghers syndrome and sudden death.

2.1.2.1.2 Lipid-rich Sertoli cell tumour (Fig. 109)

A Sertoli cell tumour in which the cytoplasm is distended with small lipid vacuoles.

This type of tumour corresponds to similar ovarian tumours.

2.1.3 Granulosa cell tumour (Figs. 110–112)

A rare testicular tumour identical to the granulosa cell tumour of the ovary.

Two types are recognized: the adult and the juvenile. Both display the same histological patterns as their ovarian counterparts.

2.1.3.1 Adult type granulosa cell tumour (Fig. 110)

The nuclei are vesicular and grooved, but they may be large, round and hyperchromatic. The cells are small, round or hexagonal; the cytoplasm is generally scant. The tumour may have a diffuse or microfollicular pattern with Call-Exner bodies. About half of the patients have gynaecomastia.

2.1.3.2 Juvenile type granulosa cell tumour (Figs. 111–112)

These cells are polyhedral or round and contain abundant pale to eosinophilic cytoplasm. The nuclei are round or oval and hyperchromatic with occasional nucleoli. There may be many mitoses. Histologically, the tumour is usually cystic but may be follicular or have solid areas. The follicles are usually large and round, oval or irregular and contain basophilic or eosinophilic fluid which is mucicarmine positive. The solid areas show sheets, nodules or irregular tubules. The tumour is almost always encountered before the age of two years. It is the most common testicular tumour of the newborn. A few have been reported in cryptorchid testes with intersex disorders.

2.1.4 Tumours of the thecoma/fibroma group (Fig. 113)

Tumours of the thecoma/fibroma group resemble their ovarian counterparts.

2.2 Incompletely differentiated sex cord/gonadal stromal tumours (Fig. 114)

Tumours composed largely of undifferentiated tissue in which abortive tubule formation, islands of Leydig cells or evidence of other specific sex cord/gonadal stromal cell types are identified.

2.3 Mixed forms

Tumours with combinations of differentiated sex cord/gonadal stromal cell types, e. g. Sertoli and Leydig cell tumours.
    These occur mainly in AIS. The components should be specified.

2.4 Unclassified forms

Sex cord/gonadal stromal tumours that do not fall into any defined category (Fig. 115).
    The criteria for malignancy of all sex cord/gonadal stromal tumours are discussed under Sect. 2.1.1.

3 Tumours Containing Both Germ Cell and Sex Cord/Gonadal Stromal Elements (Figs. 116–119)

Two categories are recognized:

3.1 Gonadoblastoma (Figs. 116–117)

A tumour composed of two principal cell types: large germ cells similar to those of seminoma and small cells resembling immature Sertoli and granulosa cells; elements resembling Leydig and lutein cells may also be present.

The two cells (germ cell and sex cord/gonadal stromal elements) are usually in irregular or rounded discrete nests, presenting one or more of three patterns. Most often the sex cord cells surround rounded hyaline nodules of basement membrane substance which merges with the surrounding basement membrane. The second pattern consists of nests composed of large germ cells surrounded by many smaller Sertoli cells. In the third growth pattern, the Sertoli cells form a ring of single cells at the periphery of a central nest of germ cells. Focal calcification may begin in hyaline bodies, sometimes forming large, wavy, laminated masses separated by dense fibrous tissue. Large polyhedral cells resembling Leydig cells but without Reinke crystals may be present after puberty.

Sometimes the germ cells of a gonadoblastoma transgress the margins of the nests and grow as a seminoma or embryonal carcinoma with only small foci of gonadoblastoma within them or at their margins. The type of germ cell tumour should be specified.

Gonadoblastomas arise almost exclusively in patients with rudimentary or streak gonads, most of whom are phenotypic females and almost all of whom are X-chromatin-negative and have a Y-chromosome.

3.2 Mixed germ cell – sex cord/gonadal stromal tumours, unclassified (Figs. 118–119)

A tumour consisting of closely admixed germ cells and sex cord/ gonadal stromal cells.

The germ cells resemble spermatogonia with ample cytoplasm and varying amounts of glycogen. The nuclei are round and may have nucleoli. The germ cells are seen either as single cells or small groups and grow in association with cells resembling Sertoli, granulosa and/or Leydig cells. The proportions of the constituent cells vary. Mitotic activity can occur, but the tumour appears to be benign.

In contrast to gonadoblastoma, these tumours occur in testes of normal males.

4 Miscellaneous Tumours

4.1 Carcinoid tumour (Fig. 120)

Carcinoid tumours resemble those that arise at other sites and have an insular, acinar, trabecular or mixed growth pattern. The tumour may be a component of a teratoma and should then be classified in category 1.2.7.3 and appropriately designated; however, it may occur in pure form either as a primary growth (classified here, Sect. 4.1) or as a metastasis (classified in Sect. 10, *Secondary Tumours*). The distinction between the last two can be difficult.

4.2 Tumours of ovarian epithelial types (Figs. 121–122)

Tumours of tunical surface that resemble surface epithelial tumours of the ovary.

These rare tumours include Brenner tumours; benign, borderline and malignant, serous and non-serous tumours; endometrioid carcinoma; clear cell adenocarcinoma; and tumours of mixed cell types.

5 Lymphoid and Haematopoietic Tumours

This category is applied to tumours of the haematopoietic system initially manifested as testicular tumours.

5.1 Lymphoma (Fig. 123)

The neoplastic cells are generally of B-cell lineage, but any type may occur. Although the infiltration is mainly intertubular, invasion of tubules occurs in about one-third of the cases. Such tubules almost invariably are within the tumour. Extratesticular extension is common. Hodgkin disease is extremely rare in the testis.

Lymphoma is more common in men over 60 years of age, but may occur at any age. Testicular involvement is often promptly followed by generalized disease. Bilaterality is common, but often delayed, sometimes until years later.

5.2 Plasmacytoma (Fig. 124)

This may be the initial manifestation of systemic disease or multiple myeloma. It has the same pattern of growth as other lymphomas.

5.3 Leukaemia (Fig. 125)

This is rarely initially manifested as a testicular tumour but more frequently in post-therapy relapse of leukaemia in children.

6 Tumours of Collecting Ducts and Rete

The ducts which connect the epididymis and the testis have been designated as tubuli recti, rete testis and ductuli efferentes, but in practice, the region is commonly referred to simply as "rete" or as "collecting ducts". This is appropriate as tumours in this area cannot, at the present time, be recognized as arising in one or another of these anatomic sites.

6.1 Adenoma (Figs. 126–127)

A benign epithelial tumour which may be tubulopapillary, cystic or adenofibromatous.

The cells are small and cuboidal. In atrophic testes, the rete may be quite prominent and simulate an adenoma (Fig. 128).

6.2 Carcinoma (Figs. 129–130)

A malignant epithelial tumour of rete or duct.

Carcinoma of the collecting ducts or rete may be tubular, papillary, cystic or solid. Before the diagnosis of collecting duct and rete carcinoma is accepted, a metastatic carcinoma or mesothelioma should be ruled out.

7 Tumours of the Tunica, Epididymis, Spermatic Cord, Supporting Structures, and Appendices

A variety of uncommon tumours is found in these sites. The topography of the tumour is important in determining its origin and multiple sections may be necessary. This is particularly true in lesions of the appendices.

7.1 Adenomatoid tumour (Figs. 131–133)

A benign tumour of mesothelial cells characterized by numerous gland-like spaces, clefts or cords.

The fibrous stroma is often hyalinized and there may be lymphocytic infiltrates, particularly around the periphery. Smooth muscle cells are often present. The tumour occurs in the epididymis more frequently than in the testicular capsule and spermatic cord. It may expand into the testis.

Synonym: benign mesothelioma.

7.2 Mesothelioma (Figs. 134–136)

Neoplastic proliferations of mesothelium similar to those of the abdomen occur. They may be benign or malignant, but sometimes the distinction between the two is difficult. Hyperplasias, often papillary, and sequestrations of mesothelium in inflammatory lesions can simulate neoplasms (Fig. 137).

7.3 Adenoma (Figs. 138–139)

A benign epithelial tumour forming glandular or papillary structures.

These tumours usually involve the epididymis. Among tumours of this type are those that occur in the von Hippel-Lindau syndrome. These often have a papillary component and consist of clear cells.

7.4 Carcinoma (Figs. 140–141)

A malignant epithelial tumour forming glandular or papillary structures.

This tumour can be diagnosed only when the possibility of metastatic disease is excluded.

7.5 Melanotic neuroectodermal tumour (Figs. 142–143)

A melanin-containing tumour with varying proportions of two cell types in a cellular fibrous stroma: epithelium-like cells, often arranged in strands, and small, darkly staining lymphocyte-like cells.

Melanin is found within the epithelium-like cells and to a lesser extent within the lymphocyte-like cells. The tumour arises in the epididymis and rarely in the testis.

Synonyms: retinal anlage tumour, melanotic hamartoma and melanotic progonoma.

7.6 Desmoplastic small round cell tumour (Figs. 144–146)

A malignant serosa-related small round cell tumour with an epithelial growth pattern in a desmoplastic stroma.

The tumour cells exhibit epithelial and myogenous differentiation by immunohistochemistry (keratin and desmin). The tumour involves the tunical surface of the epididymis or testis and is similar to the tumour encountered in the peritoneal cavity. It has a poor prognosis.

8 Soft Tissue Tumours (Figs. 147–150)

These are classified according to the *WHO Histological Classification of Soft Tissue Tumours*[1]. Embryonal rhabdomyosarcoma is seen particularly in infants, children and young adults. Lei-

---

[1] Weiss SW (1994) World Health Organization histological typing of soft tissue tumours, 2nd edn. Springer, Berlin Heidelberg New York

omyoma, leiomyosarcoma, lipoma, liposarcoma and malignant fibrous histiocytoma occur mainly in older patients.

9 Unclassified Tumours

These are primary, benign or malignant tumours that cannot be placed in any of the above categories.

10 Secondary Tumours (Fig. 151)

A testicular tumour may be the initial manifestation of an extragonadal malignant tumour. Small nests or aggregates of cells infiltrate the stroma of the testis, epididymis and cord with relative sparing of the tubules. In most cases, tumour cells are found in vascular and lymphatic spaces. The more common primary sites (in the order of frequency) are lung, prostate, gastrointestinal tract, pancreas, skin (melanoma), kidney and urinary bladder.

11 Tumour-Like Lesions

11.1 Nodules of immature tubules (Fig. 152)

These consist of coiled tubules lined by immature Sertoli cells. They are commonly encountered in undescended testes.

Synonyms: Sertoli cell nodule, persistent immature tubules, Pick-adenoma.

11.2 Testicular lesions of adrenogenital syndrome (Fig. 153)

A diffuse and/or nodular proliferation of large cells resembling both Leydig cells and adrenocortical cells occurring with adrenogenital syndrome.

These cells have abundant eosinophilic cytoplasm which typically contains a large amount of lipofuscin pigment, resulting in a dark colour of the gross surface. They typically have a hyaline fibrous stroma. Exceptionally, the nuclei are atypical. Mitotic figures may be present. The lesions are often bilateral. Since it is not certain if the proliferation constitutes a hyperplastic or neoplastic process, it is classified as a tumour-like lesion.

11.3 Testicular lesions in androgen insensitivity syndrome (Figs. 154–156)

Hamartomatous lesions with three components: seminiferous tubules, Leydig cells and ovarian-type stroma associated with the androgen insensitivity syndrome.

Two categories are recognized. In complete AIS, the external genitalia are unequivocally female. In the prepubertal stage, the testes are of normal size and histology and resemble normal prepubertal males. A myomatous mass may be present lateral to the testes. In adults, the seminiferous tubules are small and contain mostly Sertoli cells with few spermatogonia. Spermatogenesis is absent. The Leydig cells are hyperplastic. Several types of tumours in the sex cord/gonadal stromal category occur in the testes of AIS. The most common is a pure Sertoli tumour made up of closely packed uniform solid tubules containing immature Sertoli cells. Much less common is a Leydig cell tumour. These are generally considered hamartomatous when occurring in AIS.

The most serious complication of complete AIS is the development of a germ cell tumour, mostly seminoma (but rarely embryonal carcinoma), which is said to occur in 30% of patients after the age of 50.

In incomplete AIS, the external genitalia are ambiguous. Partial maturation of genital elements may be present. In elderly patients, hyalinization and cystic areas may be seen. Intratubular malignant germ cells have rarely been reported, but there is no increased incidence of malignant germ cell tumours in incomplete AIS.

11.4 Nodular precocious maturation (Fig. 157)

Unilateral nodular enlargement of the testes due to an imbalance in maturation of testicular components.

Varying degrees of maturation of seminiferous tubules and Leydig cells occur as ill-defined nodules with little or no maturation of adjacent testicular tissue. This lesion may be gonadotropin induced.

11.5 Specific orchitis (Figs. 158–160)

Orchitis due to a specific infectious agent.

Viral orchitis secondary to mumps is seen mostly in young adults and may be bilateral. It may precede the parotitis. In the early stages, the interstitium is oedematous followed by congestion and lymphocytic infiltration. Later interstitial haemorrhage is seen accompanied by inflammatory cell infiltration of the seminiferous tubules, degeneration of germ cells and eventual patchy hyalinization of seminiferous tubules and parenchymal scar.

Tuberculous orchitis is secondary to extension from epididymal tuberculosis. Syphilitic orchitis, however, may be confined to the body of the testis. It may occur in the secondary or in the tertiary stage. Other infections such as brucellosis, rickettsia and parasitic diseases may be mistaken for tumours.

11.6 Non-specific orchitis

Orchitis in which no aetiological organism is demonstrable.

11.7 Granulomatous orchitis (Fig. 161)

Orchitis characterized by intratubular and interstitial granulomatous inflammation of undetermined cause.

11.8 Malakoplakia (Figs. 162–163)

A granulomatous orchitis in which large histiocytes with abundant granular eosinophilic cytoplasm containing Michaelis-Gutmann bodies occupy the seminiferous tubules and interstitial tissues.

In some cases special stains, e. g. PAS, von Kossa or iron may be required to demonstrate the inclusions.

11.9 Adrenal cortical rest (Fig. 164)

These nodules show the zones seen in normal adrenal cortex and occur in the rete testis, tunica albuginea, between the epididymis and the testis, and in the spermatic cord.

11.10 Fibromatous periorchitis (Figs. 165–166)

A diffuse or focal fibroblastic proliferation, often hyalinized, in tunica albuginea and/or spermatic cord.

Most cases present as multiple hyalinized nodules.

Synonyms: fibromatous pseudotumour, chronic proliferative periorchitis, pseudofibromatous periorchitis, nodular periorchitis.

11.11 Funiculitis

A primary inflammation of the spermatic cord.

11.12 Residua of meconium peritonitis (Fig. 167)

A foreign body granulomatous reaction with cellular and mucinous debris and epithelial cells with or without calcification.

11.13 Sperm granuloma (Fig. 168)

A granulomatous lesion, usually in the epididymis or spermatic cord, resulting from the extravasation of spermatozoa.

This occurs in the cord following vasectomy. There are numerous phagocytes containing spermatozoa which are sometimes calcified.

11.14 Vasitis nodosa (Fig. 169)

A proliferation of small tubular or gland-like structures penetrating the muscular coat of the vas deferens and usually associated with sperm granulomas. It usually develops after vasectomy.

11.15 Sclerosing lipogranuloma (Fig. 170)

A reactive sclerosing lesion due to the injection of oily material, characterized by a granulomatous and fibrotic reaction.
It may simulate liposarcoma.

11.16 Gonadal splenic fusion (Fig. 171)

The abnormality occurs in two forms: continuous and discontinuous. In the continuous form, a cord connects the spleen to the testis by multiple small nodules of ectopic splenic tissue; whereas, in the discontinuous form, no cord is present. The left testis is almost invariably involved.

11.17 Mesonephric remnants (Fig. 172)

Residual glomeruli and renal tubules occasionally become hyperplastic and form a tumour-like lesion. Nephroblastoma in this location is believed to arise from such remnants.

11.18 Endometriosis

Paratesticular endometriosis occurs in patients after prolonged oestrogen treatment.

11.19 Epidermal cyst (Fig. 173)

A cyst lined by keratinized squamous epithelium without skin appendages.

The cyst contains keratohyalin material. The lining may be eroded in some areas resulting in a foreign body giant cell reaction. If the cyst is adjacent to a scar or a focus of a recognized type of tissue, it should be classified as a teratoma. If it occurs alone, it should be classified as an epidermal cyst.

Synonym: epidermoid cyst.

11.20 Cystic dysplasia (Figs. 174–175)

Multiple anastomosing cysts of varying sizes and shapes lined by a single layer of flat or cuboidal epithelial cells.

This rare lesion occurs in infants and children. It may be bilateral and associated with ipsilateral renal agenesis or bilateral renal dysplasia. The process begins in the region of the rete and extends into the parenchyma which can be compressed to a thin rim.

11.21 Mesothelial cyst

11.22 Others

Other lesions that may simulate tumours are supernumerary testis; intratesticular haemorrhage; spermatocele; nodules of Leydig cells in the spermatic cord; müllerian rests; adnexal cysts of müllerian or wolffian origin; reactive hyperplasia of mesothelial cells; necrotizing or granulomatous vasculitis; epididymitis; and sarcoidosis.

TNM Classification of Tumours of the Testis[1]

(ICD-O C62)

Rules for Classification

The classification applies only to germ cell tumours of the testis. There should be histological confirmation of the disease and division of cases by histological type. Histopathological grading is not applicable.

The presence of elevated serum tumour markers, including alphafetoprotein (aFP), human chorionic gonadotropin (hCG), and lactic dehydrogenase (LDH), is frequent in this disease. Staging is based on the determination of the anatomic extent of disease and assessment of serum tumour markers.

The following are the procedures for assessing N, M, and S categories:

N categories	Physical examination and imaging
M categories	Physical examination, imaging, and biochemical tests
S categories	Serum tumour markers

Stages are subdivided based on the presence and degree of elevation of serum tumour markers. Serum tumour markers are obtained immediately after orchiectomy and, if elevated, should be performed serially after orchiectomy according to the normal decay for aFP (half-life 7 days) and hCG (half-life 3 days) to assess for serum tumour marker elevation. The S classification is based on the nadir value of hCG and aFP after orchiectomy. The serum level of LDH (but not its half-life levels) has prognostic value in patients with metastatic disease and is included for staging.

---

[1] Sobin LH, Wittekind Ch (eds) (1997) TNM classification of malignant tumours, 5th ed. Wiley, New York

Regional Lymph Nodes

The regional lymph nodes are the abdominal para-aortic (peri-aortic), preaortic, interaortocaval, precaval, paracaval, retrocaval and retroaortic nodes. Nodes along the spermatic vein should be considered regional. Laterality does not affect the N classification. The intrapelvic nodes and the inguinal nodes are considered regional after scrotal or inguinal surgery.

TNM Clinical Classification

T – Primary tumour

The extent of the primary tumour is classified after radical orchiectomy; see pT. If no radical orchiectomy has been performed, TX is used.

N – Regional Lymph Nodes

NX   Regional lymph nodes cannot be assessed
N0   No regional lymph node metastasis
N1   Metastasis with a lymph node mass 2 cm or less in greatest dimension or multiple lymph nodes, none more than 2 cm in greatest dimension
N2   Metastasis with a lymph node mass more than 2 cm but not more than 5 cm in greatest dimension, or multiple lymph nodes, any one mass more than 2 cm but not more than 5 cm in greatest dimension
N3   Metastasis with a lymph node mass more than 5 cm in greatest dimension

M – Distant Metastasis

MX   Distant metastasis cannot be assessed
M0   No distant metastasis
M1   Distant metastasis
    M1a   Non-regional lymph node or pulmonary metastasis
    M1b   Distant metastasis other than to non-regional lymph nodes and lungs

pTNM Pathological Classification

pT – Primary Tumour

pTX Primary tumour cannot be assessed (if no radical orchiectomy has been performed TX is used)

pT0 No evidence of primary tumour (e.g. histologic scar in
testis)

pTis Intratubular germ cell neoplasia (carcinoma in situ)

pT1 Tumour limited to testis and epididymis without vascular/
lymphatic invasion; tumour may invade tunica albuginea
but not tunica vaginalis.

pT2 Tumour limited to testis and epididymis with vascular/
lymphatic invasion, or tumour extending through tunica
albuginea with involvement of tunica vaginalis.

pT3 Tumour invades spermatic cord with or without vascular/
lymphatic invasion.

pT4 Tumour invades scrotum with or without vascular/lympha-
tic invasion.

pN – Regional Lymph Nodes

pNX Regional lymph nodes cannot be assessed

pN0 No regional lymph node metastasis

pN1 Metastasis with a lymph node mass 2 cm or less in greatest
dimension and 5 or fewer positive nodes, none more than
2 cm in greatest dimension

pN2 Metastasis with a lymph node mass more than 2 cm but
not more than 5 cm in greatest dimension; or more than
5 nodes positive, none more than 5 cm; or evidence of
extranodal extension of tumour

pN3 Metastasis with a lymph node mass more than 5 cm in
greatest dimension

pM – Distant Metastasis

The pM category corresponds to the M category.

S – Serum Tumour Markers

SX   Serum marker studies not available or not performed
S0   Serum marker study levels within normal limits

	LDH		**hCG(mIU/ml)**		**aFP (ng/ml)**
S1	$< 1.5 \times N$	and	$< 5,000$	and	$< 1,000$
S2	$1.5–10 \times N$	or	$5,000–50,000$	or	$1,000–10,000$
S3	$> 10 \times N$	or	$> 50,000$	or	$> 10,000$

N indicates the upper limit of normal for the LDH assay

Stage Grouping

Stage 0	pTis	N0	M0	S0,SX
Stage I	pT1–4	N0	M0	SX
Stage IA	pT1	N0	M0	S0
Stage IB	pT2	N0	M0	S0
	pT3	N0	M0	S0
	pT4	N0	M0	S0
Stage IS	Any pT/TX	N0	M0	S1–3
Stage II	Any pT/TX	N1–3	M0	SX
Stage IIA	Any pT/TX	N1	M0	S0
	Any pT/TX	N1	M0	S1
Stage IIB	Any pT/TX	N2	M0	S0
	Any pT/TX	N2	M0	S1
Stage IIC	Any pT/TX	N3	M0	S0
	Any pT/TX	N3	M0	S1
Stage III	Any pT/TX	Any N	M1, M1a	SX
Stage IIIA	Any pT/TX	Any N	M1, M1a	S0
	Any pT/TX	Any N	M1, M1a	S1
Stage IIIB	Any pT/TX	N1–3	M0	S2
	Any pT/TX	Any N	M1, M1a	S2
Stage IIIC	Any pT/TX	N1–3	M0	S3
	Any pT/TX	Any N	M1, M1a	S3
	Any pT/TX	Any N	M1b	Any S

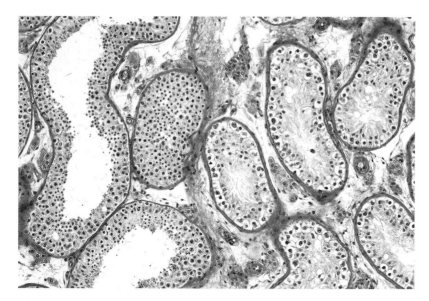

Fig. 1. *Intratubular malignant germ cells*

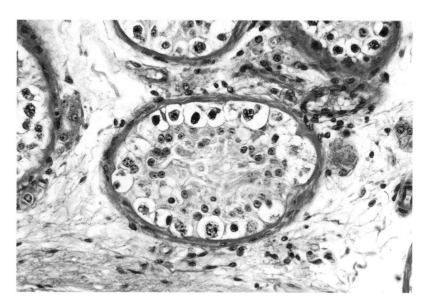

Fig. 2. *Intratubular malignant germ cells*

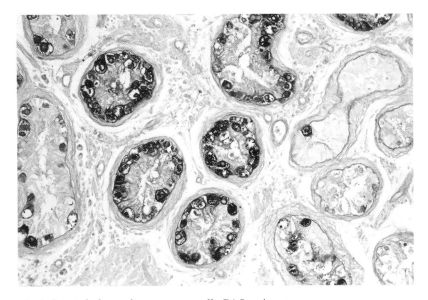

Fig. 3. *Intratubular malignant germ cells.* PAS stain

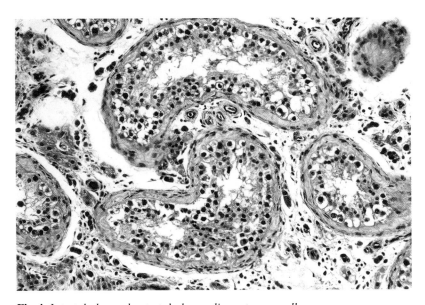

Fig. 4. *Intratubular and extratubular malignant germ cells*

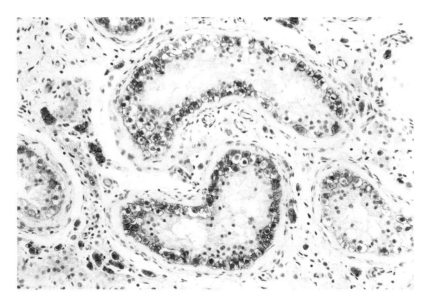

Fig. 5. *Intratubular and extratubular malignant germ cells.* Anti-PLAP, same field as Fig. 4

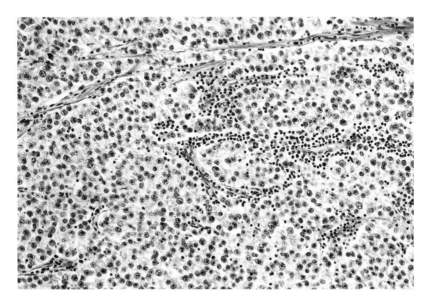

Fig. 6. *Seminoma*

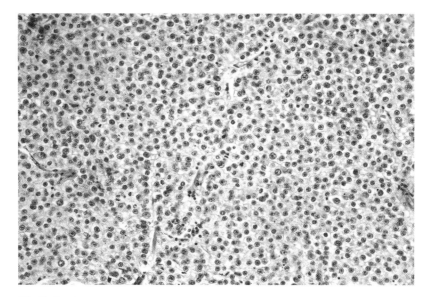

Fig. 7. *Seminoma*

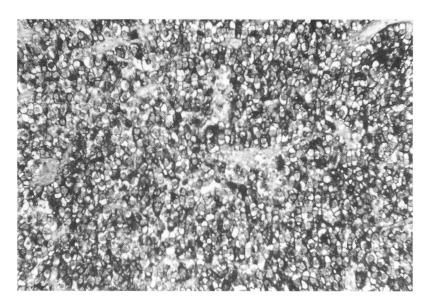

Fig. 8. *Seminoma.* PAS stain

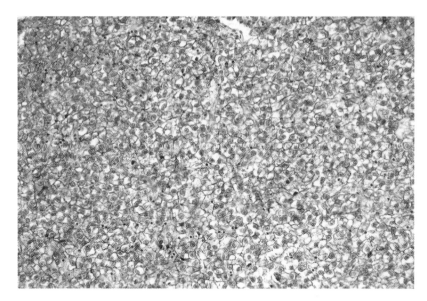

Fig. 9. *Seminoma.* anti-PLAP

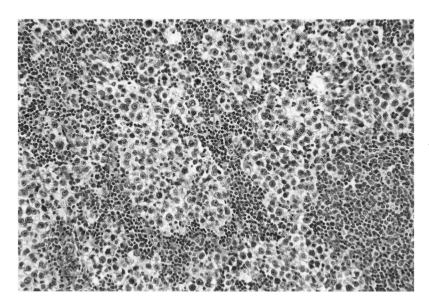

Fig. 10. *Seminoma.* Lymphocytic infiltration

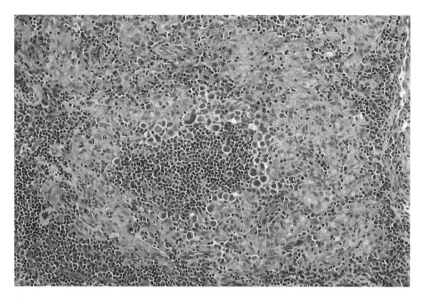

Fig. 11. *Seminoma.* Granulomatous reaction

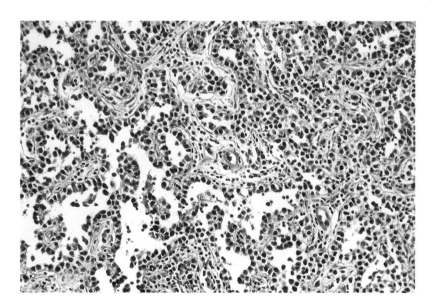

Fig. 12. *Seminoma.* Alveolar pattern

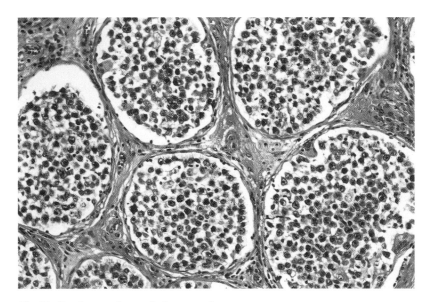

Fig. 13. *Seminoma.* Intratubular growth pattern

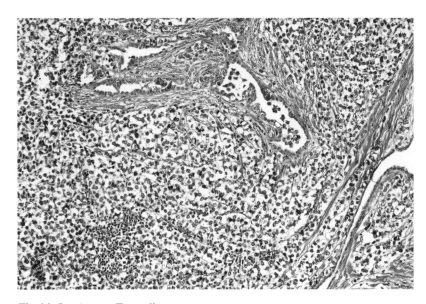

Fig. 14. *Seminoma.* Extending to rete

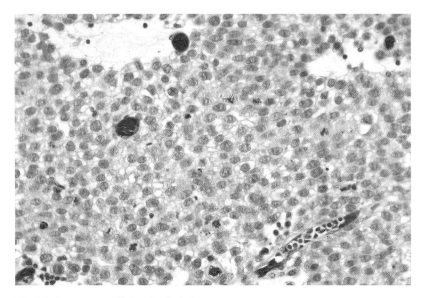

Fig. 15. *Seminoma.* High mitotic index

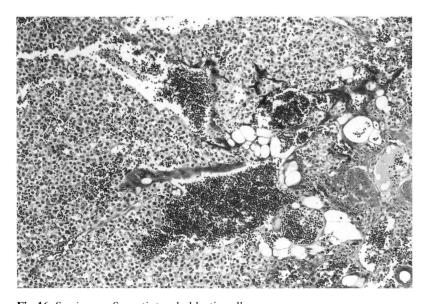

Fig. 16. *Seminoma.* Syncytiotrophoblastic cells

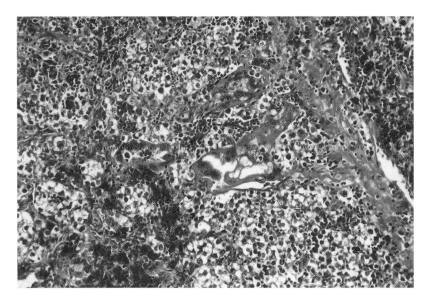

Fig. 17. *Seminoma.* Syncytiotrophoblastic cells associated with haemorrhage

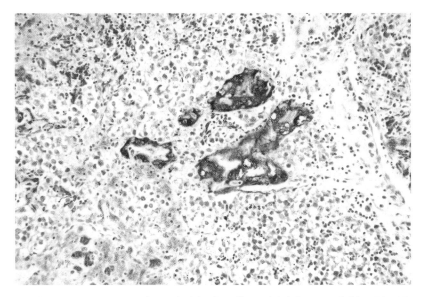

Fig. 18. *Seminoma.* Syncytiotrophoblastic cells, anti-hCG, same field as Fig. 17

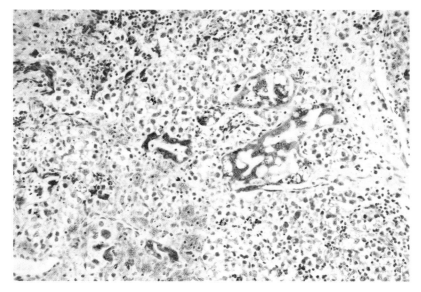

Fig. 19. *Seminoma.* Syncytiotrophoblastic cells, anti-hPL, same field as Fig. 17

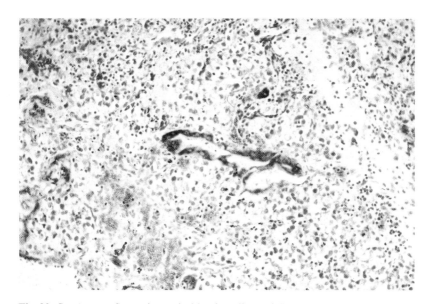

Fig. 20. *Seminoma.* Syncytiotrophoblastic cells, anti-SP1, same field as Fig. 17

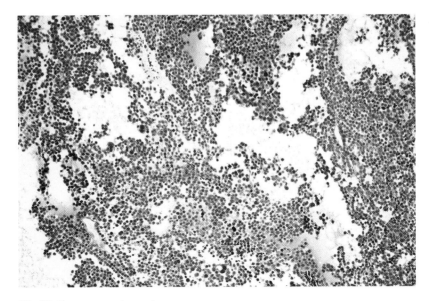

Fig. 21. *Spermatocytic seminoma*

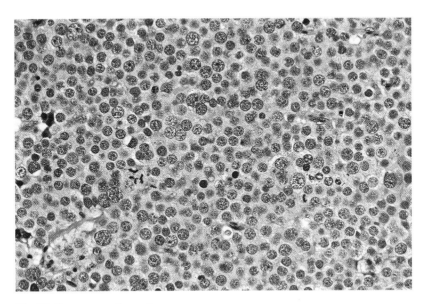

Fig. 22. *Spermatocytic seminoma*

50

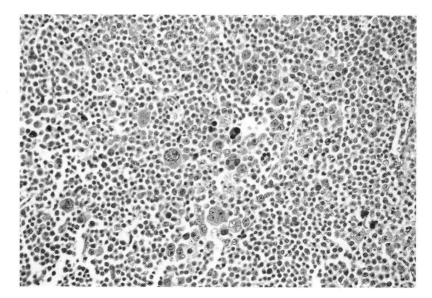

Fig. 23. *Spermatocytic seminoma*

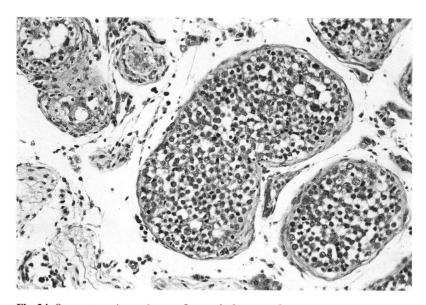

Fig. 24. *Spermatocytic seminoma.* Intratubular growth pattern

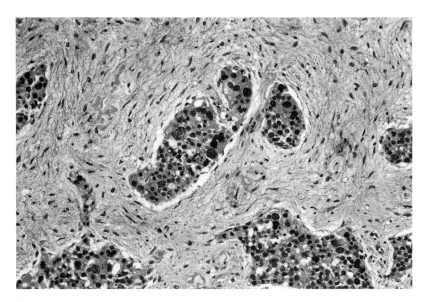

Fig. 25. *Spermatocytic seminoma with sarcoma*

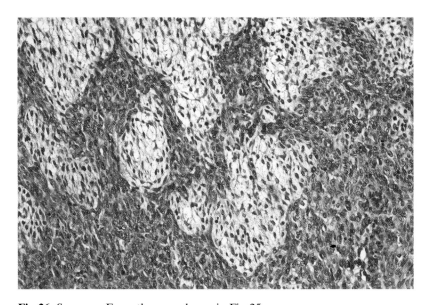

Fig. 26. *Sarcoma.* From the case shown in Fig. 25

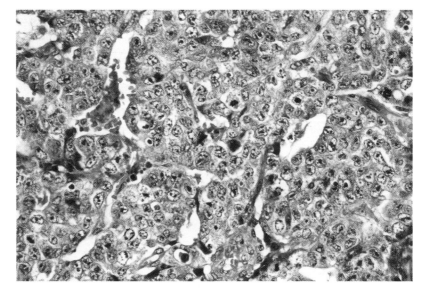

Fig. 27. *Embryonal carcinoma.* Solid pattern

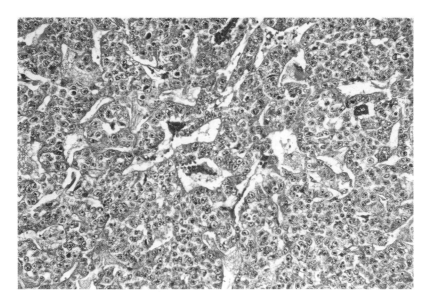

Fig. 28. *Embryonal carcinoma.* Solid and tubular patterns

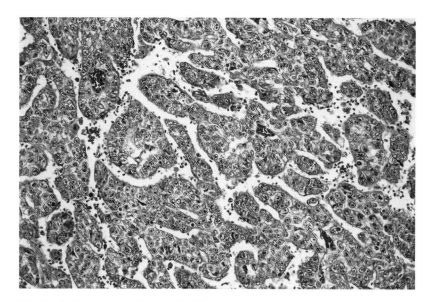

Fig. 29. *Embryonal carcinoma.* Papillary pattern

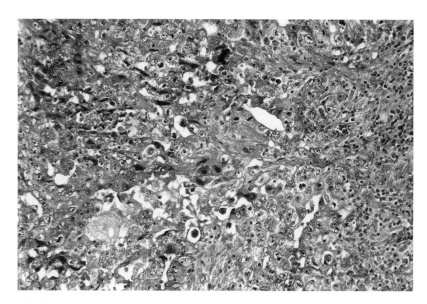

Fig. 30. *Embryonal carcinoma*

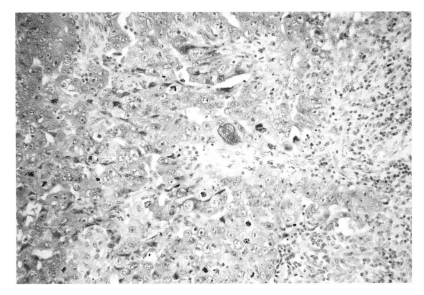

Fig. 31. *Embryonal carcinoma.* Anti-aFP, same field as Fig. 30

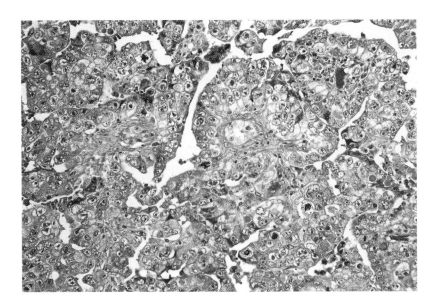

Fig. 32. *Embryonal carcinoma*

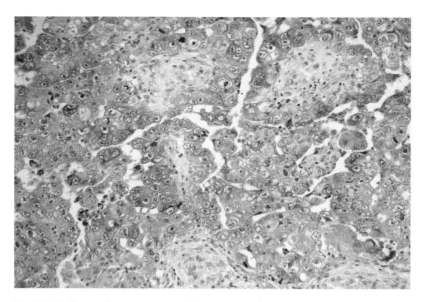

Fig. 33. *Embryonal carcinoma.* Anti-hPL, same field as Fig. 32

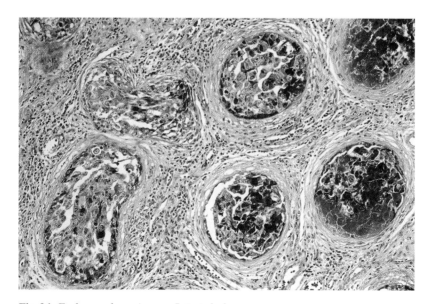

Fig. 34. *Embryonal carcinoma.* Intratubular

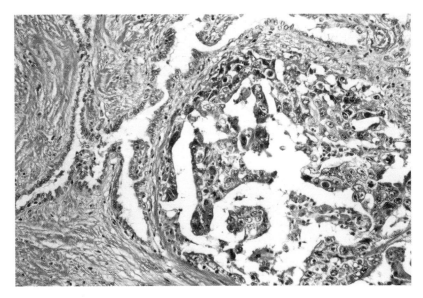

Fig. 35. *Embryonal carcinoma.* Extending to rete testis

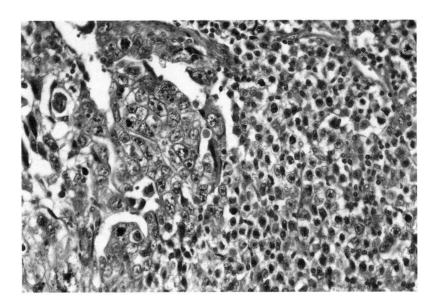

Fig. 36. *Embryonal carcinoma and seminoma*

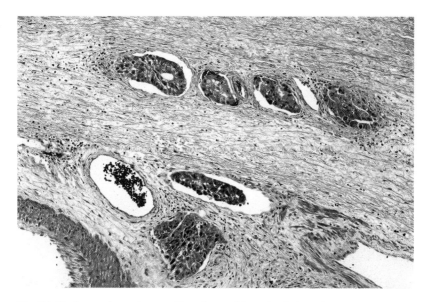

Fig. 37. *Embryonal carcinoma.* Vascular and lymphatic invasion

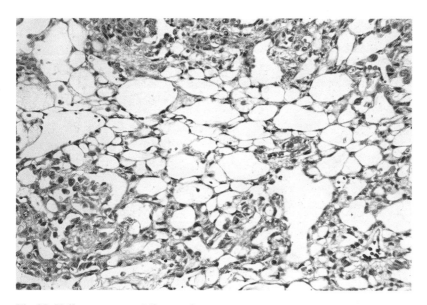

Fig. 38. *Yolk sac tumour.* Microcystic pattern

58

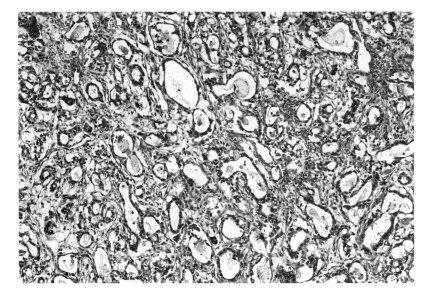

Fig. 39. *Yolk sac tumour.* Tubulo-alveolar pattern

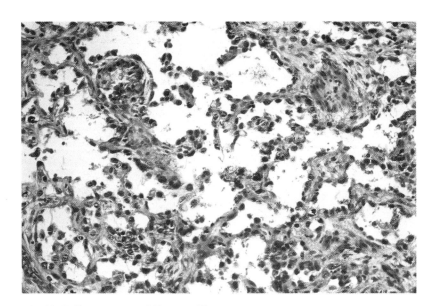

Fig. 40. *Yolk sac tumour.* Micropapillary pattern

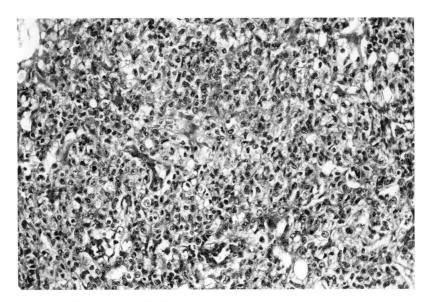

Fig. 41. *Yolk sac tumour.* Solid pattern

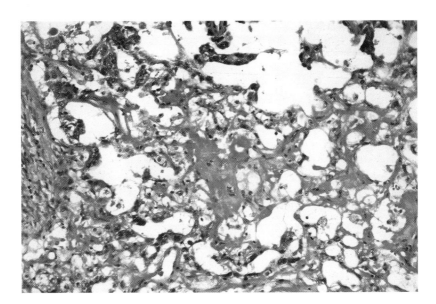

Fig. 42. *Yolk sac tumour.* Parietal pattern

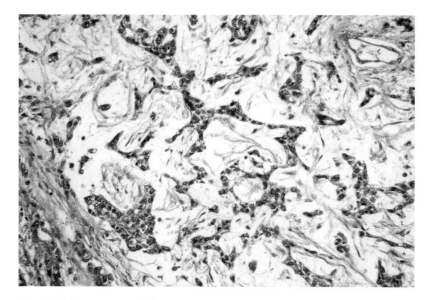

Fig. 43. *Yolk sac tumour.* Myxomatous stroma

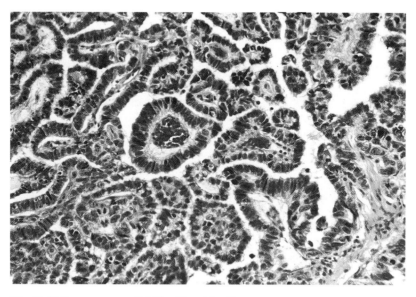

Fig. 44. *Yolk sac tumour.* Schiller-Duval bodies

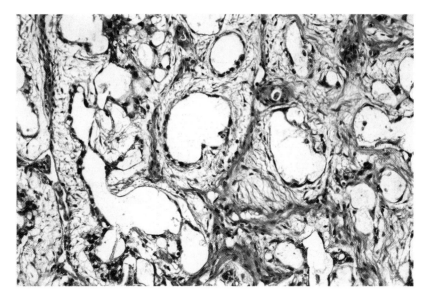

Fig. 45. *Yolk sac tumour.* Polyvesicular vitelline pattern

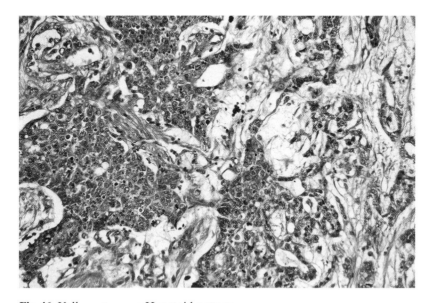

Fig. 46. *Yolk sac tumour.* Hepatoid pattern

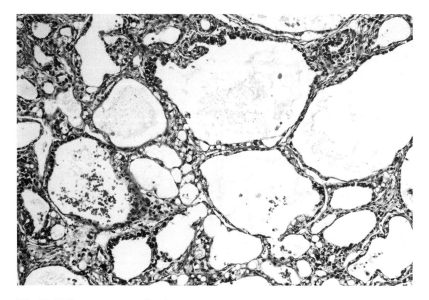

Fig. 47. *Yolk sac tumour.* Cystic pattern

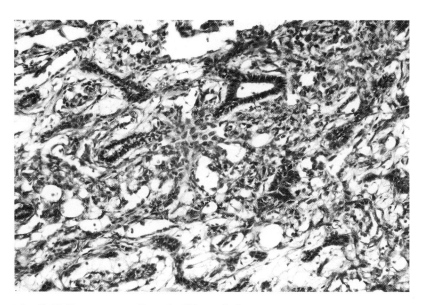

Fig. 48. *Yolk sac tumour.* Enteric differentiation

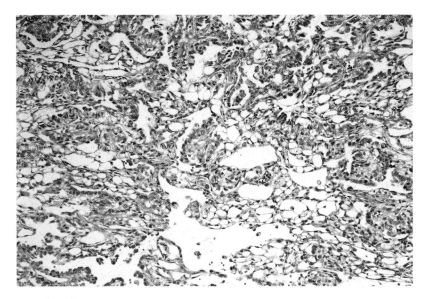

Fig. 49. *Yolk sac tumour*

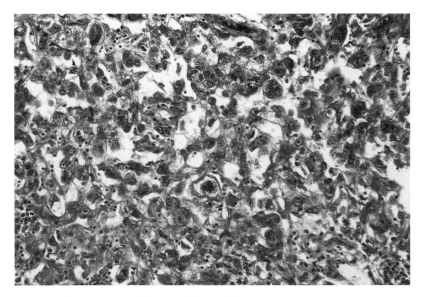

Fig. 50. *Yolk sac tumour.* Pleomorphic nuclei

64

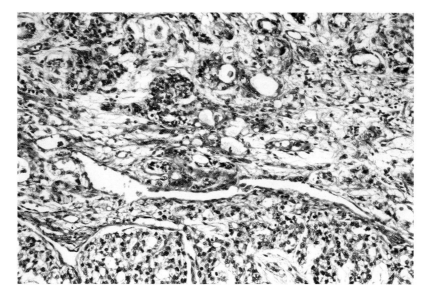

Fig. 51. *Yolk sac tumour.* Reticular pattern

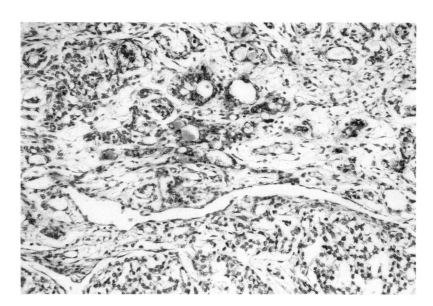

Fig. 52. *Yolk sac tumour.* Anti-aFP, same field as Fig. 51

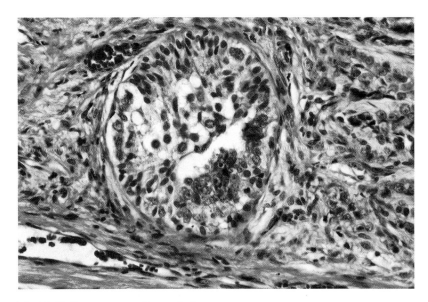

Fig. 53. *Yolk sac tumour.* Intratubular

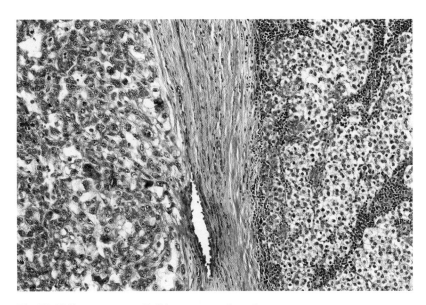

Fig. 54. *Yolk sac tumour.* Solid pattern and seminoma

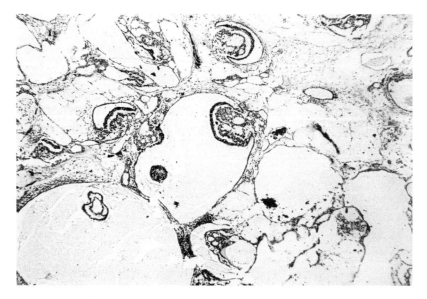

Fig. 55. *Polyembryoma.* Myxoid stroma

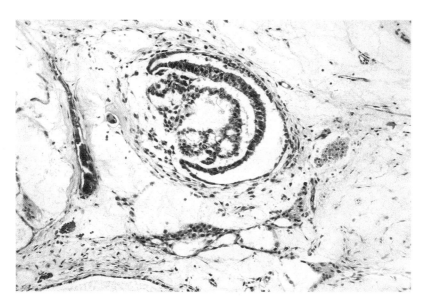

Fig. 56. *Polyembryoma.* Embryoid body

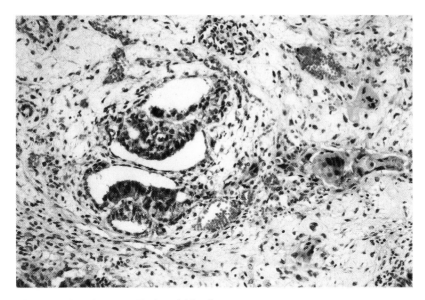

Fig. 57. *Polyembryoma.* Embryoid bodies

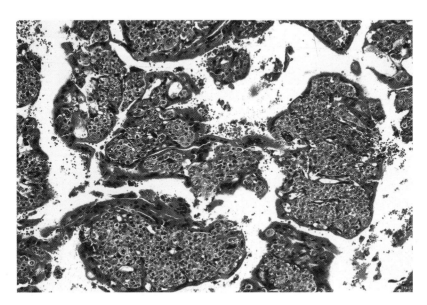

Fig. 58. *Choriocarcinoma*

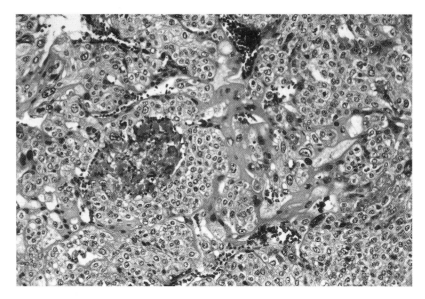

Fig.59. *Choriocarcinoma*

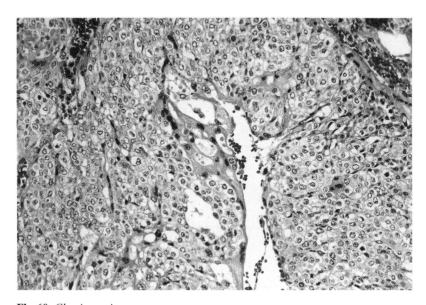

Fig.60. *Choriocarcinoma*

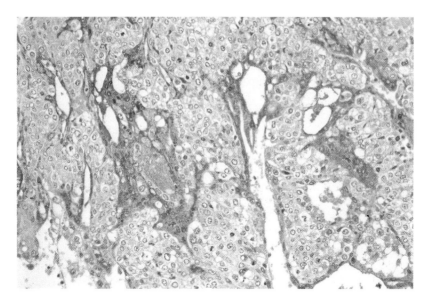

Fig. 61. *Choriocarcinoma.* Anti-hCG, same field as Fig. 60

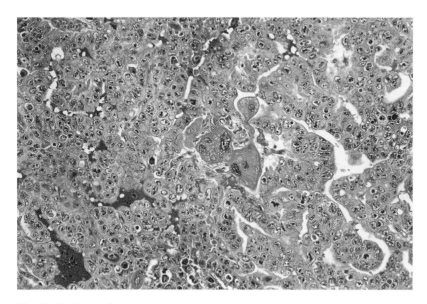

Fig. 62. *Embryonal carcinoma and syncytiotrophoblastic cells*

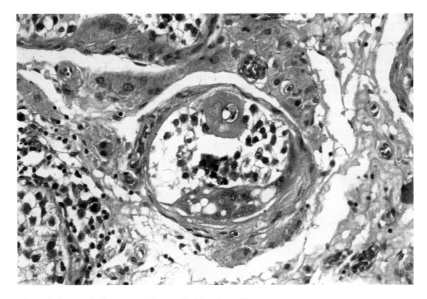

Fig. 63. *Intratubular syncytiotrophoblastic cells*

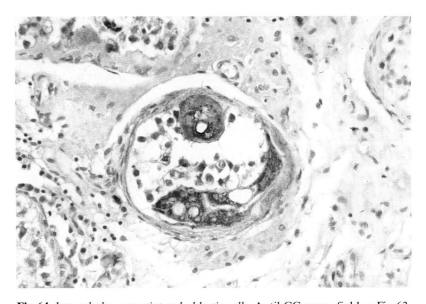

Fig. 64. *Intratubular syncytiotrophoblastic cells.* AntihCG, same field as Fig. 63

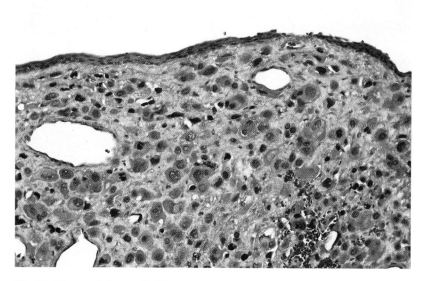

Fig. 65. *Placental site trophoblastic tumour*

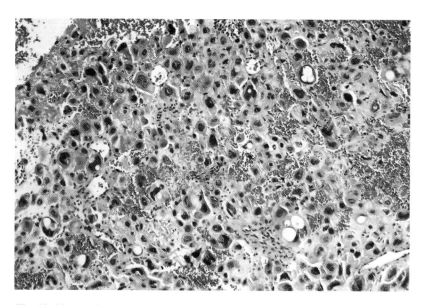

Fig. 66. *Placental site trophoblastic tumour*

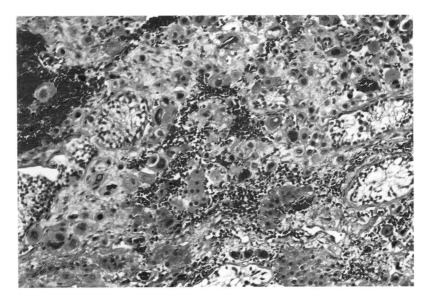

Fig. 67. *Placental site trophoblastic tumour*

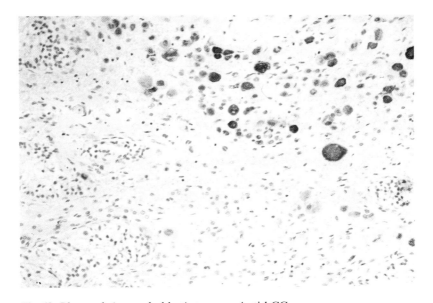

Fig. 68. *Placental site trophoblastic tumour.* Anti-hCG

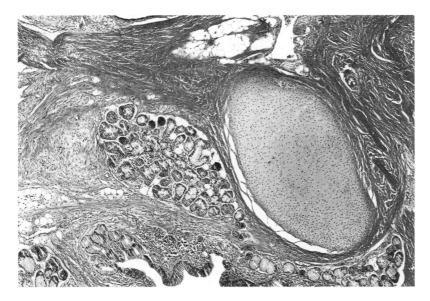

Fig. 69. *Mature teratoma*

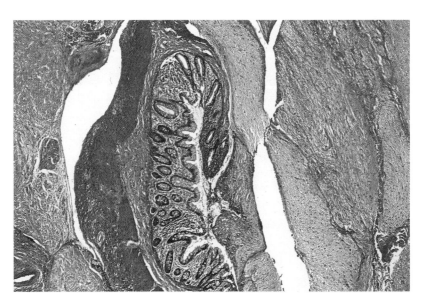

Fig. 70. *Mature teratoma*

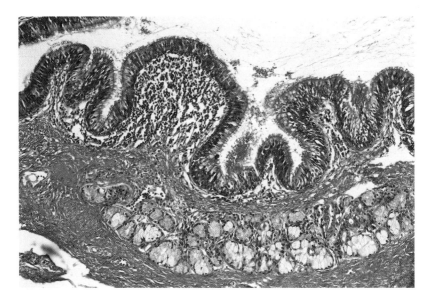

Fig. 71. *Mature teratoma*

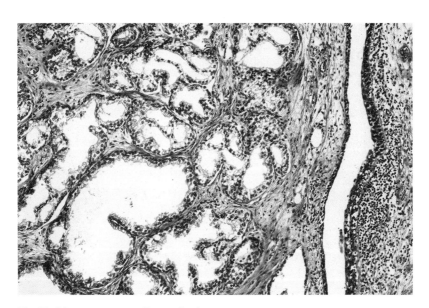

Fig. 72. *Mature teratoma.* Prostatic tissue

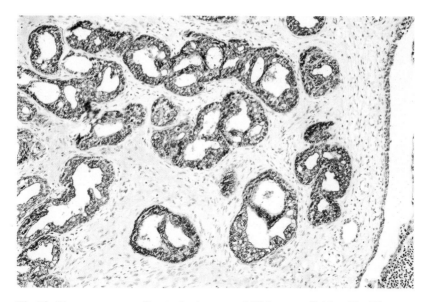

Fig. 73. *Mature teratoma.* Prostatic tissue, anti-PSA, same field as Fig. 72

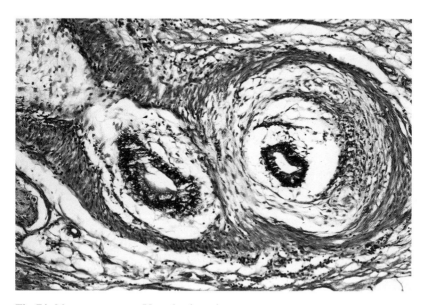

Fig. 74. *Mature teratoma.* Vascular invasion

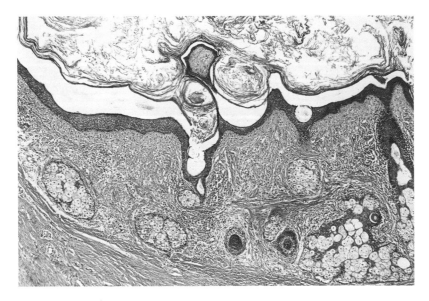

Fig. 75. *Dermoid cyst*

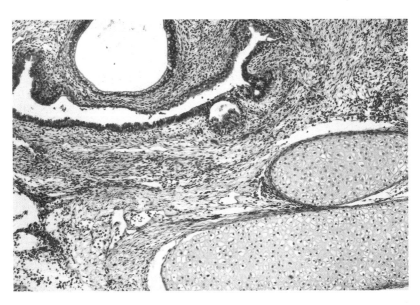

Fig. 76. *Immature teratoma*

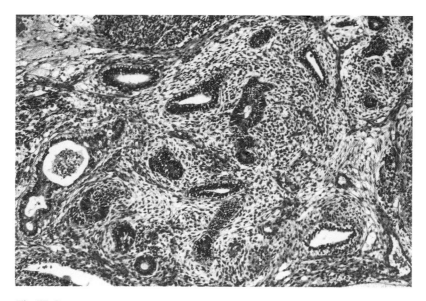

Fig. 77. *Immature teratoma*

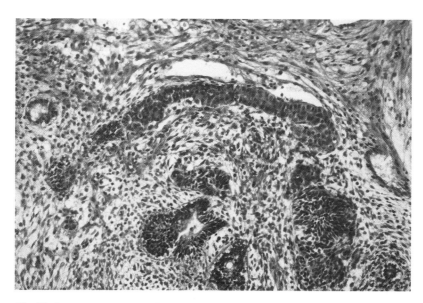

Fig. 78. *Immature teratoma.* Immature gastrointestinal glands and hepatoid differentiation

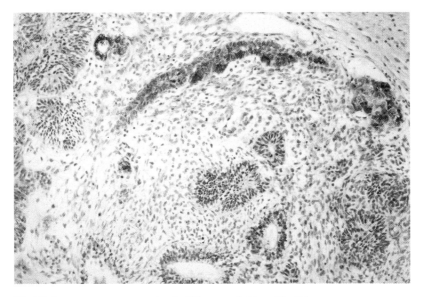

Fig. 79. *Immature teratoma.* Anti-aFP, same field as Fig. 78

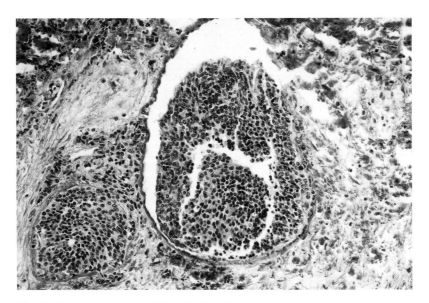

Fig. 80. *Immature teratoma.* Vascular invasion

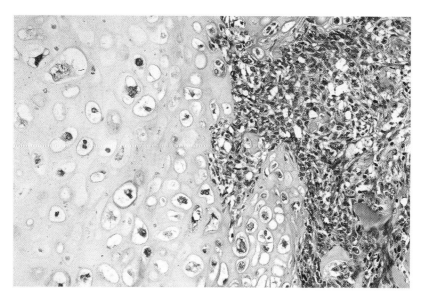

Fig. 81. *Teratoma with malignant areas.* Chondrosarcoma

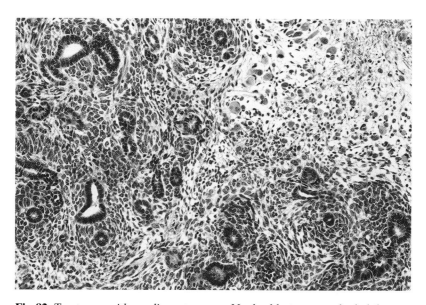

Fig. 82. *Teratoma with malignant areas.* Nephroblastoma and rhabdomyo-sarcoma

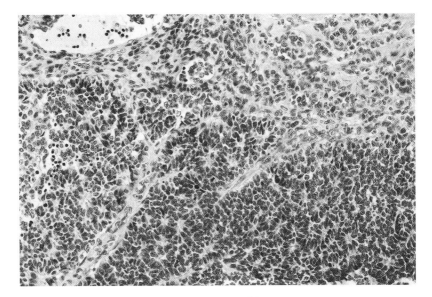

Fig. 83. *Teratoma with malignant areas.* Neuroblastoma

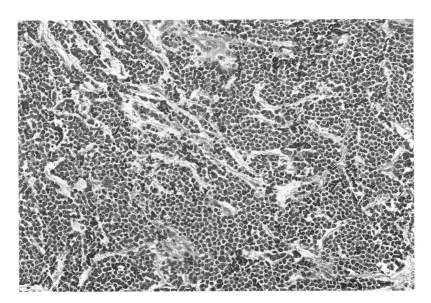

Fig. 84. *Teratoma with malignant areas.* Malignant neuroectodermal tumour

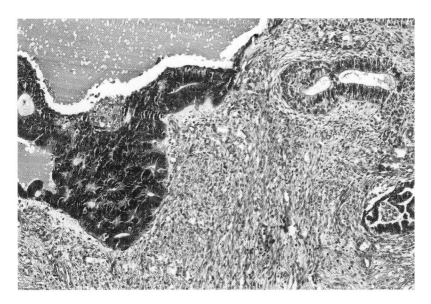

Fig. 85. *Teratoma with malignant areas.* Adenocarcinoma

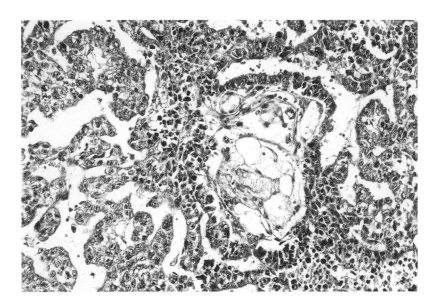

Fig. 86. *Embryonal carcinoma and yolk sac tumour*

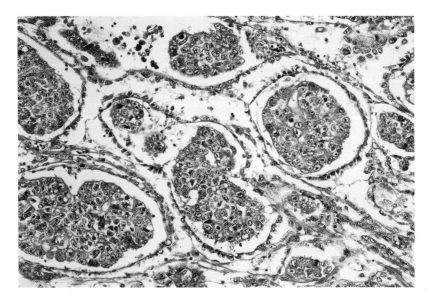

Fig. 87. *Embryonal carcinoma and yolk sac tumour*

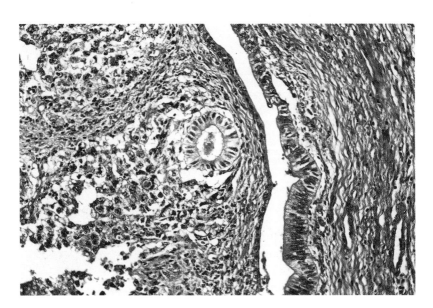

Fig. 88. *Embryonal carcinoma and teratoma*

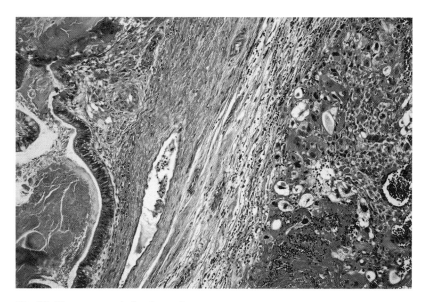

Fig. 89. *Teratoma and choriocarcinoma*

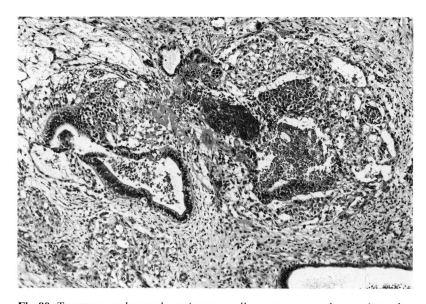

Fig. 90. *Teratoma, embryonal carcinoma, yolk sac tumour and syncytiotropho-blastic cells*

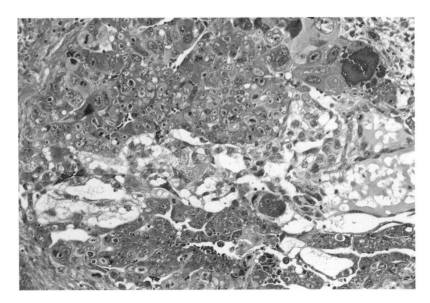

Fig. 91. *Embryonal carcinoma, yolk sac tumour and syncytiotrophoblastic cells*

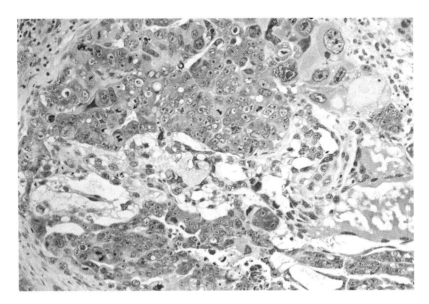

Fig. 92. *Anti-aFP,* same field as Fig. 91

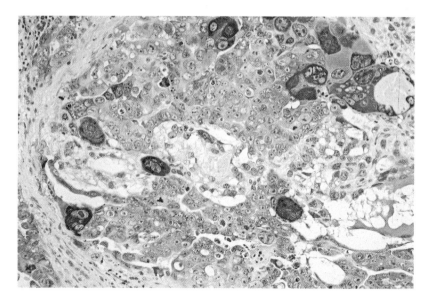

Fig. 93. *Anti-hCG,* same field as Fig. 91

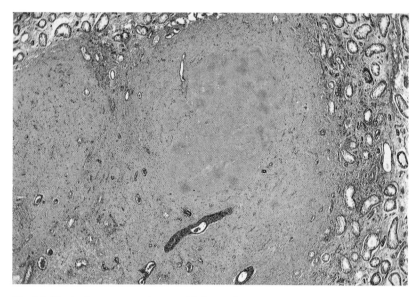

Fig. 94. *Testicular scar consistent with burned-out tumour*

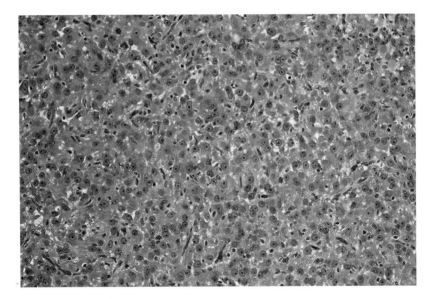

Fig. 95. *Leydig cell tumour*

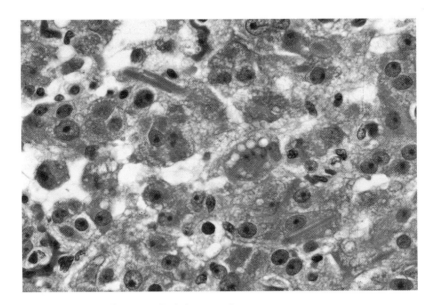

Fig. 96. *Leydig cell tumour.* Reinke crystals

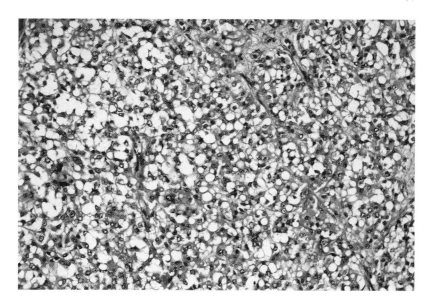

Fig. 97. *Leydig cell tumour*

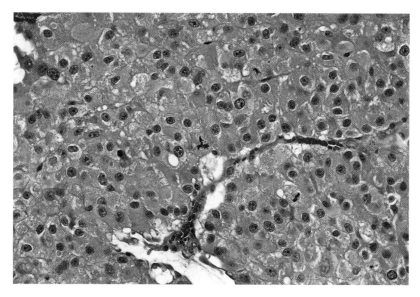

Fig. 98. *Malignant Leydig cell tumour.* Abnormal mitoses

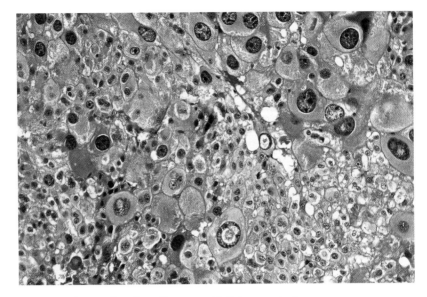

Fig. 99. *Malignant Leydig cell tumour.* Cellular anaplasia

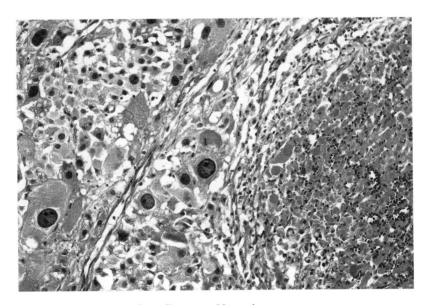

Fig. 100. *Malignant Leydig cell tumour.* Necrosis

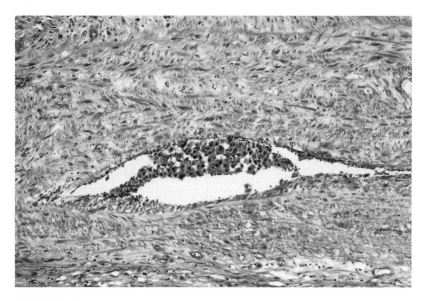

Fig. 101. *Malignant Leydig cell tumour.* Vascular invasion

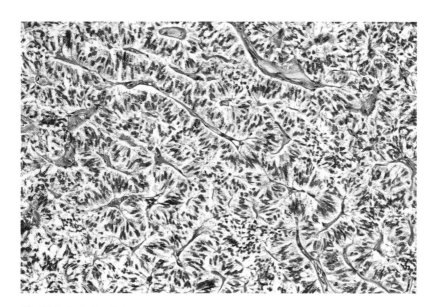

Fig. 102. *Sertoli cell tumour*

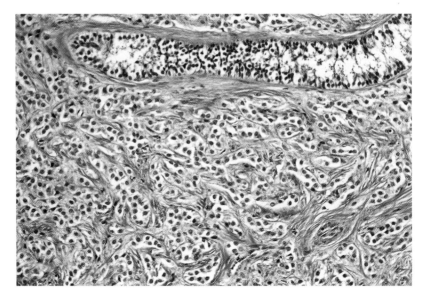

Fig. 103. *Sertoli cell tumour*

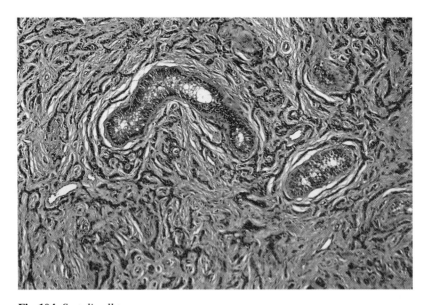

Fig. 104. *Sertoli cell tumour*

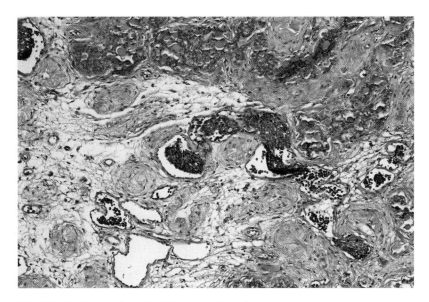

Fig. 105. *Malignant Sertoli cell tumour.* Vascular invasion

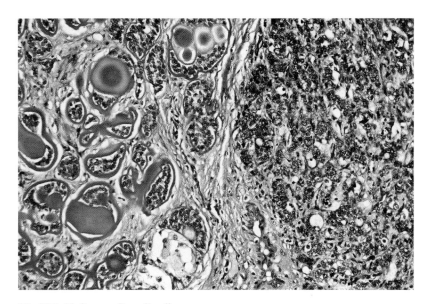

Fig. 106. *Malignant Sertoli cell tumour*

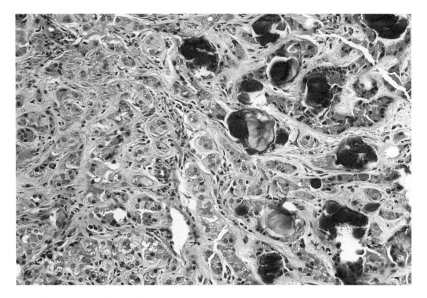

Fig. 107. *Large cell calcifying Sertoli cell tumour*

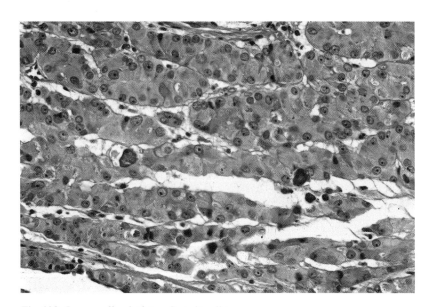

Fig. 108. *Large cell calcifying Sertoli cell tumour*

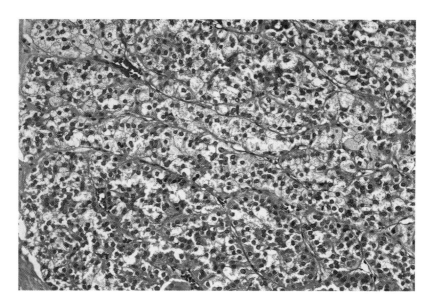

Fig. 109. *Sertoli cell tumour.* Lipid-rich type

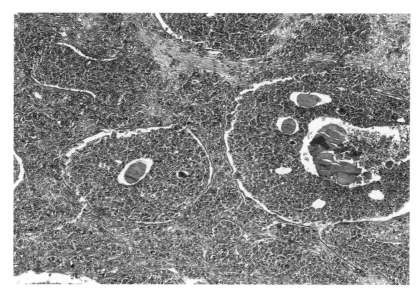

Fig. 110. *Granulosa cell tumour.* Adult type

94

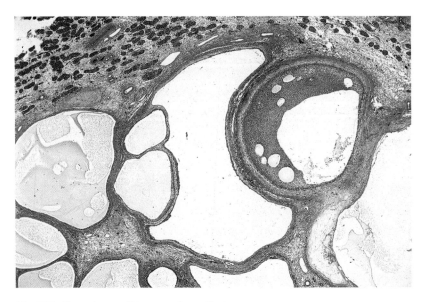

Fig. 111. *Granulosa cell tumour.* Juvenile type

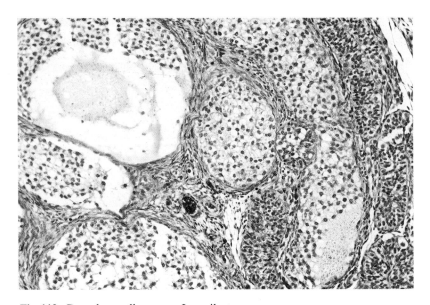

Fig. 112. *Granulosa cell tumour.* Juvenile type

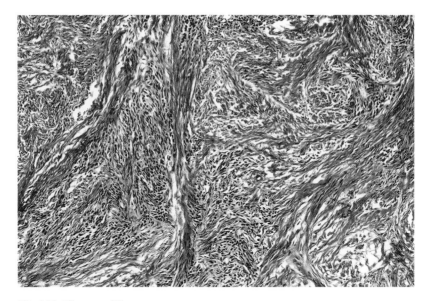

Fig. 113. *Thecoma/fibroma tumour*

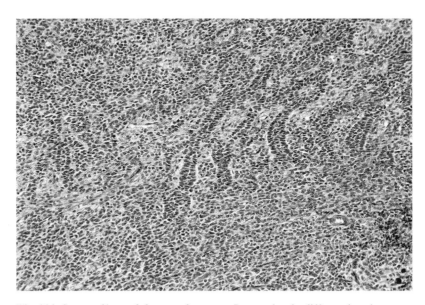

Fig. 114. *Sex cord/gonadal stromal tumour.* Incompletely differentiated

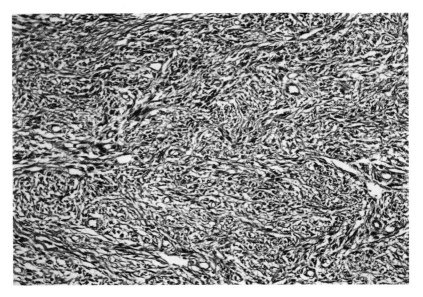

Fig. 115. *Sex cord/gonadal stromal tumour.* Unclassified form

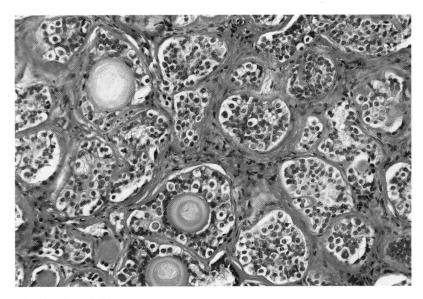

Fig. 116. *Gonadoblastoma*

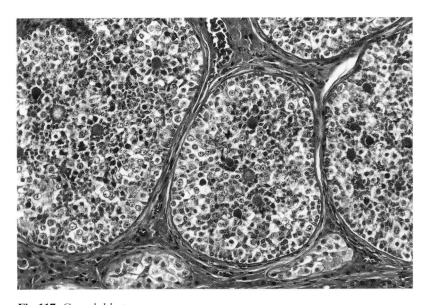

Fig. 117. *Gonadoblastoma*

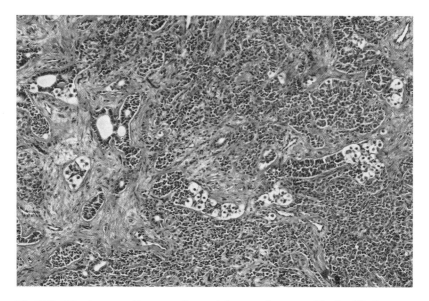

Fig. 118. *Mixed germ cell sex cord/gonadal stromal tumour.* Unclassified

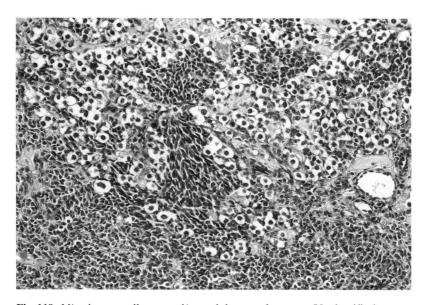

Fig. 119. *Mixed germ cell sex cord/gonadal stromal tumour.* Unclassified

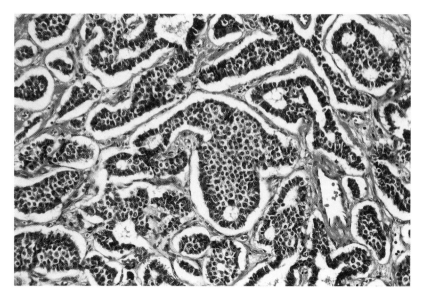

Fig. 120. *Carcinoid*

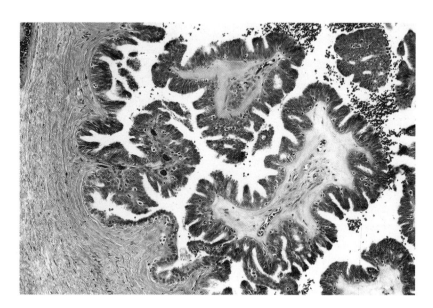

Fig. 121. *Papillary serous cystadenoma*

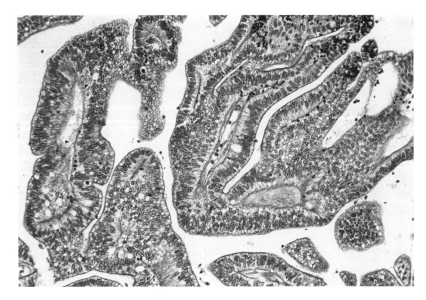

Fig. 122. *Endometrioid carcinoma*

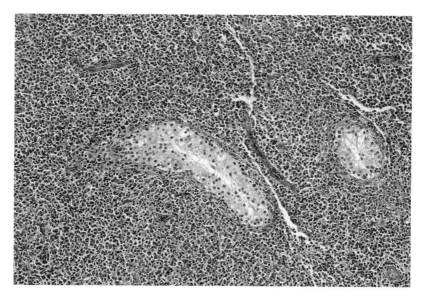

Fig. 123. *Lymphoma*

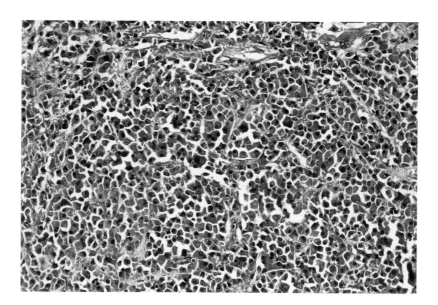

Fig. 124. *Plasmacytoma*

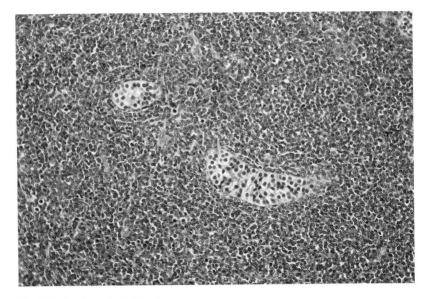

Fig. 125. *Leukaemic infiltration*

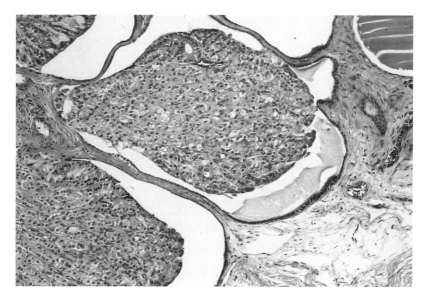

Fig. 126. *Adenoma of rete*

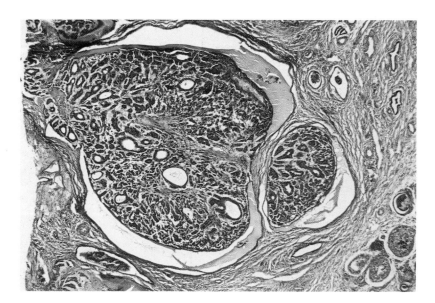

Fig. 127. *Adenoma of rete*

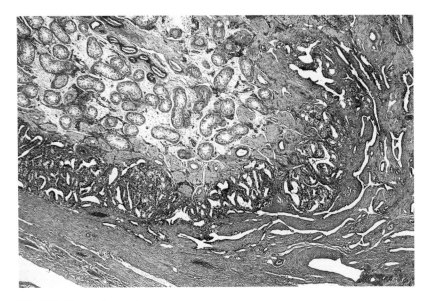

Fig. 128. *Hyperplasia of rete*

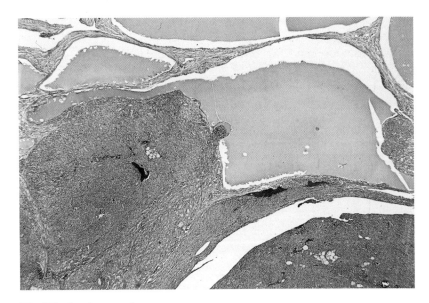

Fig. 129. *Carcinoma of rete*

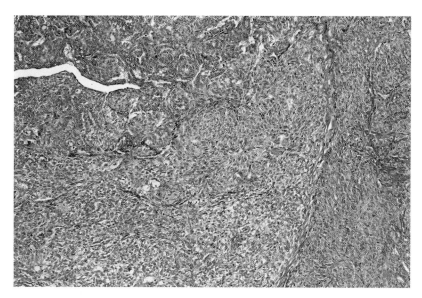

Fig. 130. *Carcinoma of rete.* Same case as Fig. 129

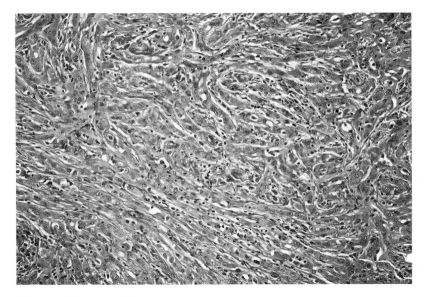

Fig. 131. *Adenomatoid tumour*

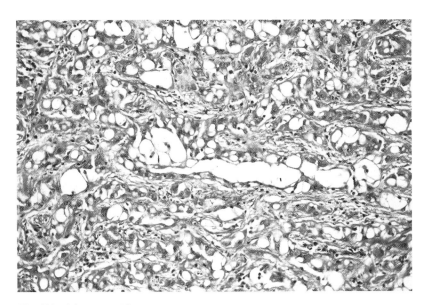

Fig. 132. *Adenomatoid tumour*

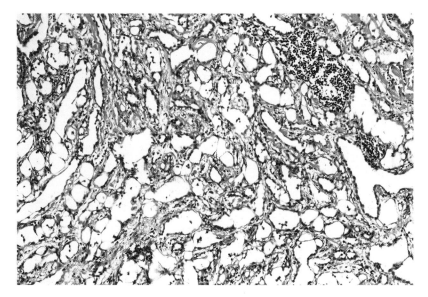

Fig. 133. *Adenomatoid tumour*

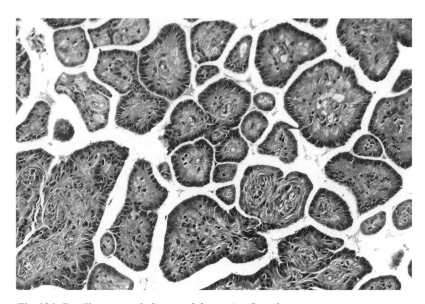

Fig. 134. *Papillary mesothelioma of the tunica.* Local recurrence

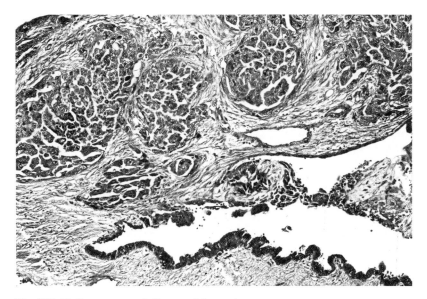

Fig. 135. *Malignant mesothelioma of the tunica*

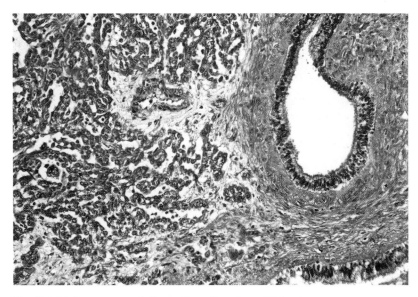

Fig. 136. *Malignant mesothelioma.* Invading the epididymis

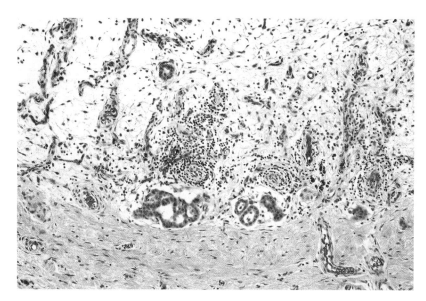

Fig. 137. *Reactive mesothelial hyperplasia*

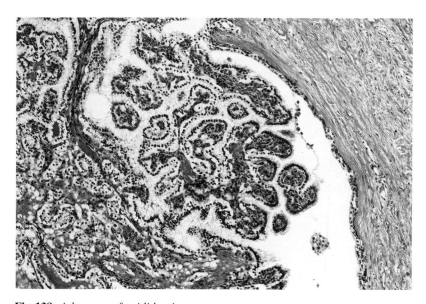

Fig. 138. *Adenoma of epididymis*

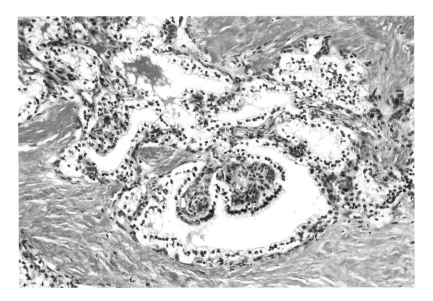

Fig. 139. *Adenoma of epididymis.* von Hippel-Lindau disease

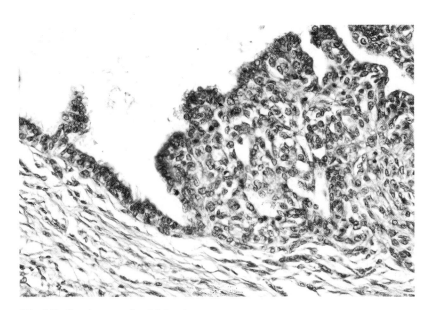

Fig. 140. *Carcinoma of epididymis*

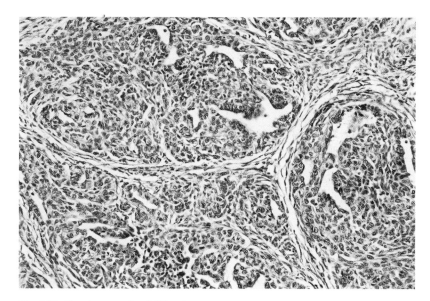

Fig. 141. *Carcinoma of epididymis*

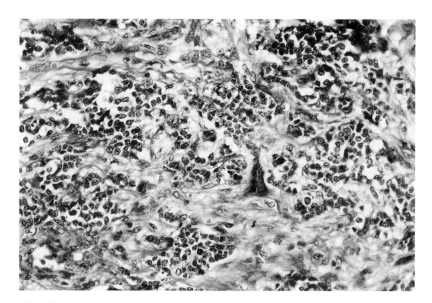

Fig. 142. *Melanotic neuroectodermal tumour*

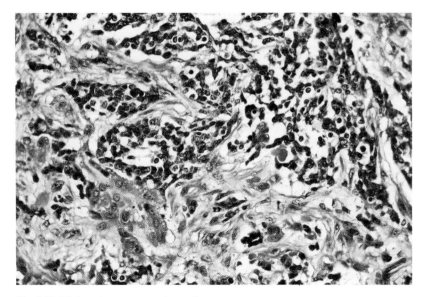

Fig. 143. *Melanotic neuroectodermal tumour*

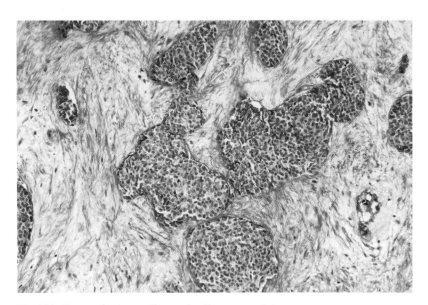

Fig. 144. *Desmoplastic small round cell tumour of the tunica*

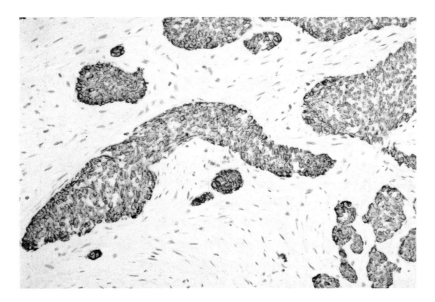

Fig. 145. *Desmoplastic small round cell tumour.* Anti-Keratin

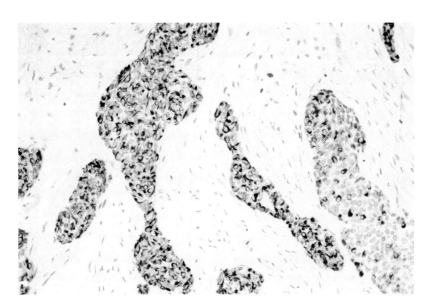

Fig. 146. *Desmoplastic small round cell tumour.* Anti-Desmin

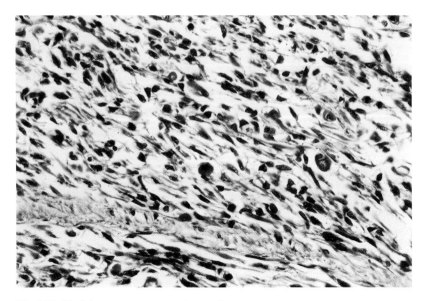

Fig. 147. *Rhabdomyosarcoma,* embryonal

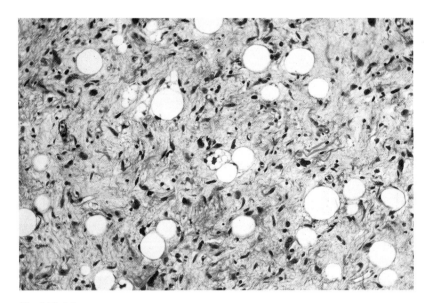

Fig. 148. *Liposarcoma*

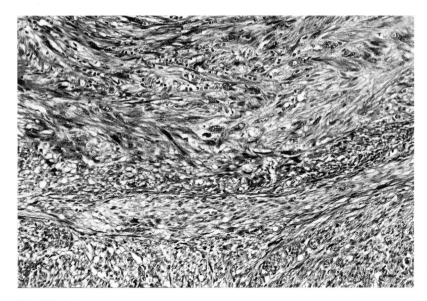

Fig. 149. *Leiomyosarcoma*

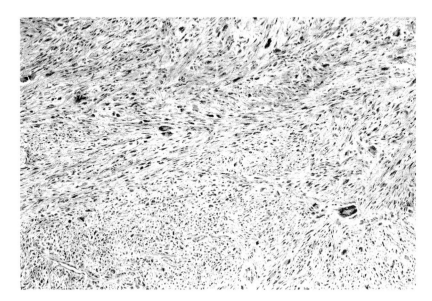

Fig. 150. *Malignant fibrous histiocytoma*

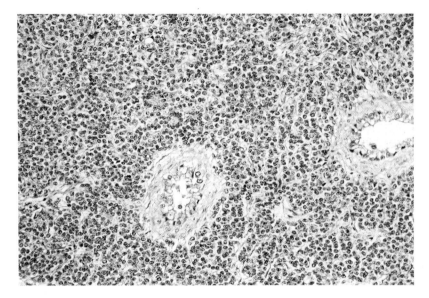

Fig. 151. *Metastatic prostatic carcinoma*

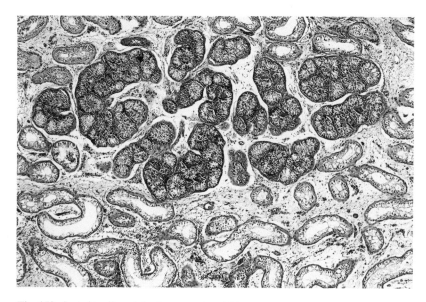

Fig. 152. *Sertoli cell nodule.* In a cryptorchid

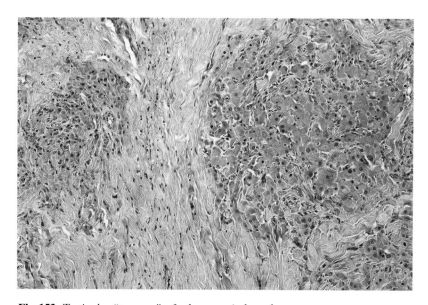

Fig. 153. *Testicular "tumour" of adrenogenital syndrome*

118

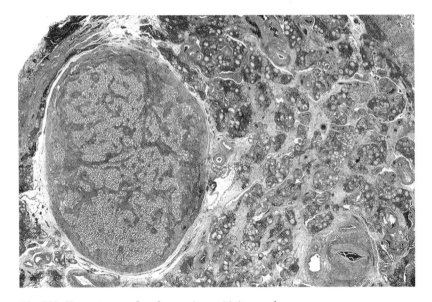

Fig. 154. *Hamartoma of androgen insensitivity syndrome*

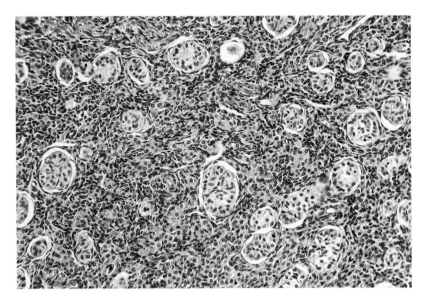

Fig. 155. *Hamartoma of androgen insensitivity syndrome.* Seminiferous tubules, Leydig cells and ovarian type stroma

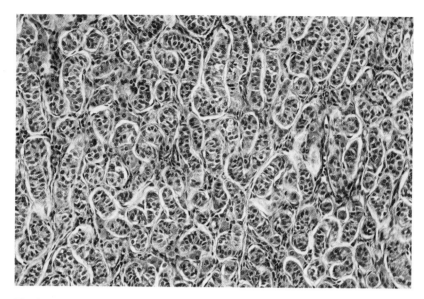

Fig. 156. *Hamartoma of androgen insensitivity syndrome.* Sertoli cell nodule

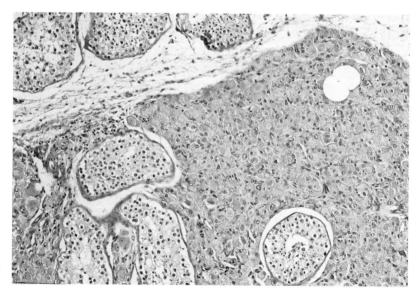

Fig. 157. Nodular precocious maturation

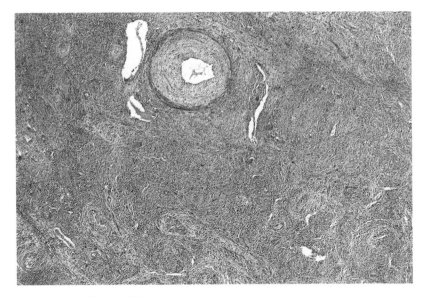

Fig. 158. *Syphilitic orchitis*

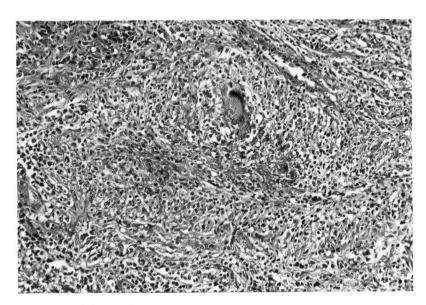

Fig. 159. *Syphilitic orchitis*

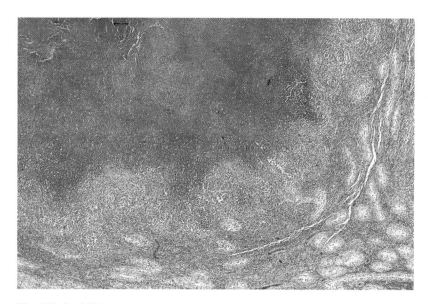

Fig. 160. *Syphilitic gumma*

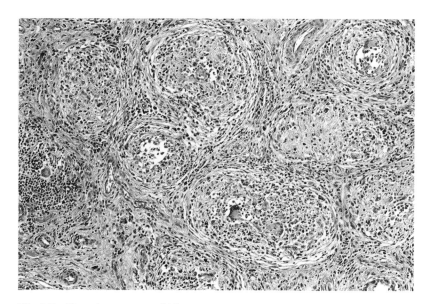

Fig. 161. *Granulomatous orchitis*

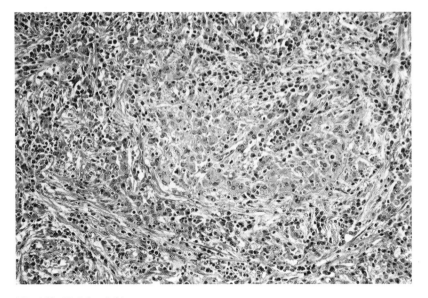

Fig. 162. *Malakoplakia*

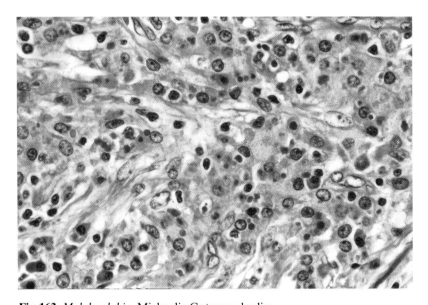

Fig. 163. *Malakoplakia.* Michaelis-Gutmann bodies

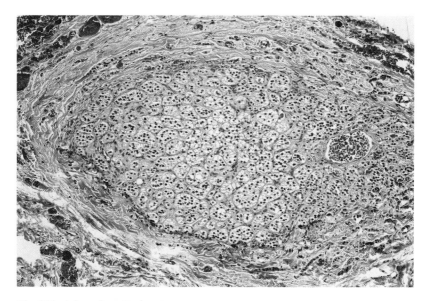

Fig. 164. *Adrenal cortical rest*

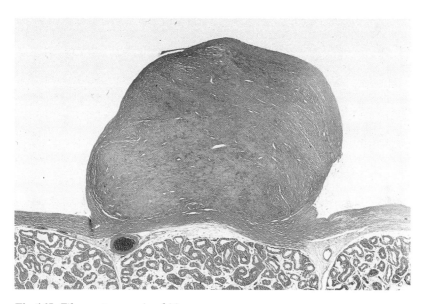

Fig. 165. *Fibromatous periorchitis*

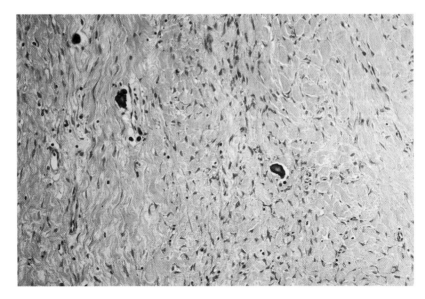

Fig. 166. *Fibromatous periorchitis*

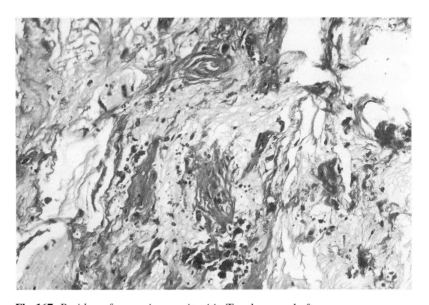

Fig. 167. *Residua of meconium peritonitis.* Two lanugo shafts

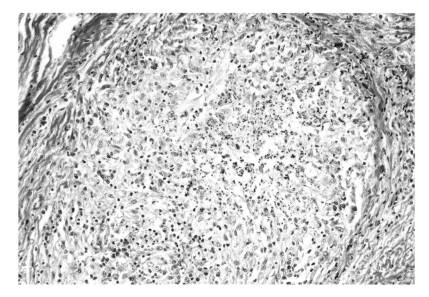

Fig. 168. *Sperm granuloma*

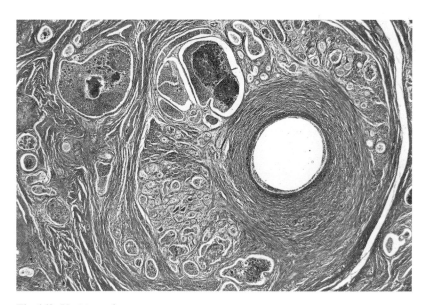

Fig. 169. *Vasitis nodosa*

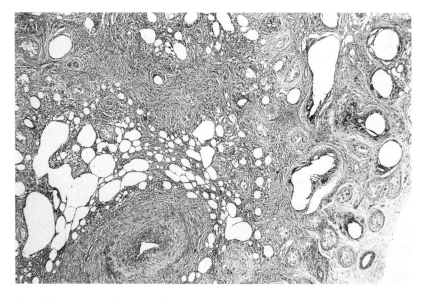

Fig. 170. *Sclerosing lipogranuloma*

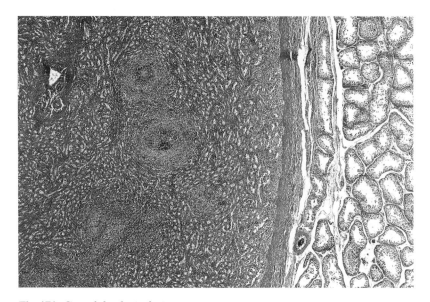

Fig. 171. *Gonadal splenic fusion*

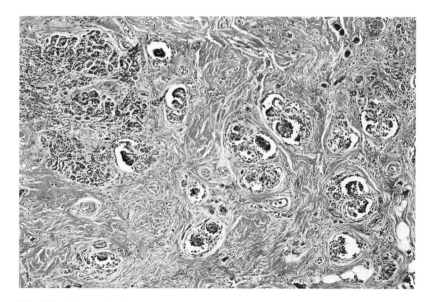

Fig. 172. *Mesonephric remnants*

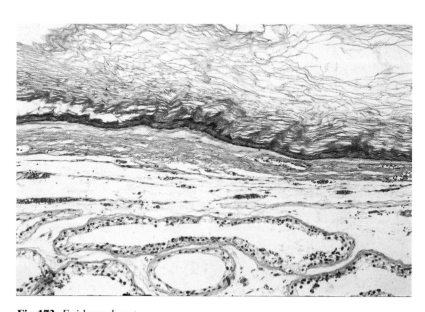

Fig. 173. *Epidermal cyst*

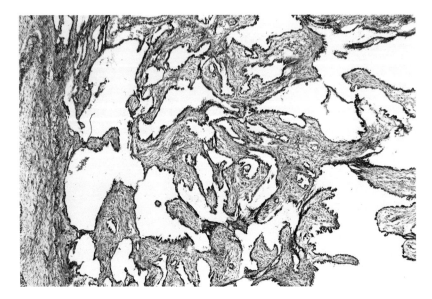

Fig. 174. *Cystic dysplasia*

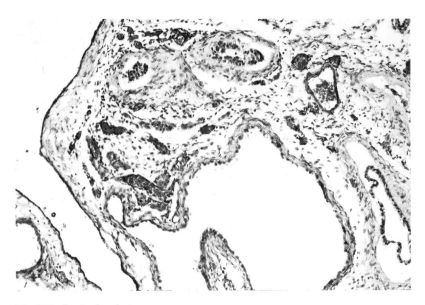

Fig. 175. *Cystic dysplasia*

Subject Index

6697620

3 1378 00669 7620